Psychiatric Hegemony

Bruce M.Z. Cohen

Psychiatric Hegemony

A Marxist Theory of Mental Illness

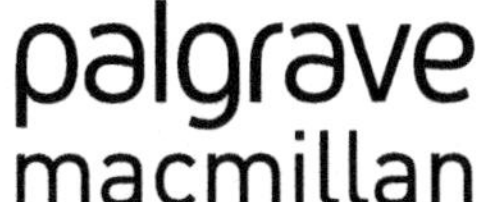

Bruce M.Z. Cohen
Department of Sociology
University of Auckland
Auckland, New Zealand

ISBN 978-1-137-46050-9 ISBN 978-1-137-46051-6 (eBook)
DOI 10.1057/978-1-137-46051-6

Library of Congress Control Number: 2016956374

Printed on acid-free paper

This Palgrave Macmillan imprint is published by Springer Nature
The registered company is Macmillan Publishers Ltd. London
The registered company address is: The Campus, 4 Crinan Street, London, N1 9XW, United Kingdom

This book is dedicated to three critical sociologists who continue to inspire:
Stanley Cohen (1942–2013)
Stuart Hall (1932–2014)
Jock Young (1942–2013)
&
An old friend and revolutionary footballer:
Hafty (d. 2014)
Es geht voran!

Preface

This book exists for two main reasons. First, to fill a gap in the current sociology of mental health scholarship. This omission was brought to my attention by my postgraduate students; though I was initially very sceptical of their research capabilities, it turned out that they were basically correct. Granted, there are bits and pieces of Marxist analysis out there, but compared with the other mainstream areas of sociological investigation such as education, youth, crime, and the family, the use of the big man's work to make sense of the continuing power of the mental health system is nearly non-existent. Second, this book offers a radical challenge to the conservative and theory-free scholarship which is currently infecting my area of sociology. I believe we need to bring critical scholarship back to the heart of the sociology of mental health; we desperately need to have the theoretical as well as the empirical debates.

The book title may suggest radical polemic, but at the same time, I think the argument is relatively simple and straightforward, and also, I think there is plenty of evidence to support it. Under capitalism, we live in a society of fundamental inequalities defined by our relation to the means of economic production. Public or private, every institution in capitalist society is framed by these same power disparities. The dominant understandings of who we are, what is expected of us, and the limits of our behaviour are constructed and defined by the capitalist class, then reproduced through the state and institutions of civil society (e.g., the systems of education, criminal justice, and health). This is necessary for the progression and survival of capitalism. For example, we are socialised by the family, the school, and the mass media to accept social and economic disparities as natural and common sense; as the inevitable result of differential talent and competition within the marketplace, rather than class privilege and the exploitation of the majority of the population. In this respect, the mental health system is no exception. Led by the institution of psychiatry as the ultimate experts on the mind, mental health professionals are far from immune to the needs of capital. In fact, I will demonstrate in this book that the mental health system has been impressively compliant to the wishes of the ruling classes and, for that reason, has gained more power, authority, and professional jurisdiction as industrial society has developed.

While this book is centrally a theoretical interrogation of psychiatric discourse and professional power, I have also attempted to make it accessible to practitioners and non-theoreticians. I think theory is vitally important to achieving a broader understanding of human existence within this world, but I appreciate that many put more faith in the "practical solution," in being "pragmatic," and in changing the world through "doing." I think mental health practitioners—and I have met plenty over the years—are particularly prone to this view. For this reason, there are four substantive chapters in the book (on the issues of work, youth, women, and political protest) which are written with the pragmatists in mind. These apply Marxist ideas to specific issues within the field and highlight the many dangers of simply "doing" mental health work without any thought to the wider structures in which they carry out such activities. Often performed by professionals who similarly believed that they were "acting in the best interests of the patient," the history of psychiatry and its allies is littered with too many acts of violence, torture, and death to be able to write them off as aberrations or exceptions in a "progressive" and "scientific" system of health care. It can instead be seen as a regular service performed by the mental health system in support of the ruling elites.

What follows is my version of a Marxist theory of mental illness. It is only one contribution within the sociology of mental health, but nevertheless, I hope it inspires others to follow my analysis in equally challenging and critical directions. And if you want to continue the discussion, you can email me at b.cohen@auckland.ac.nz or @BmzCohen on twitter.

Acknowledgements

This book could not have happened without the emphatic support of Palgrave Macmillan; I am eternally grateful for their faith and trust in this project. In particular I would like to thank my Editors, Nicola Jones and Sharla Plant, as well as the ever-helpful Assistant Editors, Eleanor Christie, Laura Aldridge and Cecilia Ghidotti. The idea for the book originated from my postgraduate "Sociology of Mental Health" class. I thank all of the students that I have had the pleasure to teach on that course over the years, in particular Dhakshi Gamage (a student who articulated the specific connection between neoliberal values and the construction of shyness as a mental disorder long before I did). In 2015 I had the chance to meet with a number of international colleagues working on critical issues in mental health and I would like to thank them all for their kind words of support and advice. They include Suman Fernando, China Mills, and Peter Morrall. My good friend Jeff Masson has become something of a mentor, what a guy! I would like to thank both him and his family for being such warm and generous people on the many occasions that we have visited them and outstayed our welcome. The Department of Sociology at the University of Auckland continues to be the home of a vibrant crowd of collegial people who understand how important it is to have the time and resources to complete a major research project like this one—many thanks to you all. Of particular note, hello to my friend and colleague Colin Cremin, with whom I have shared some really useful conversations on the slippery subject of academic writing. And he lets me win when we play PES 2016, result! Thanks also to Helen Sword for the conversation on the ferry about scholarly writing and her very useful book *Stylish Academic Writing* (I tried, Helen!). This would be an appropriate point to add that all the ideas and attempts at style in this book are my fault alone. My thanks and appreciation to the Faculty of Arts, who approved my research and study leave in 2015; this allowed me to complete most of the writing for the book. The Faculty also funded a summer scholar, Rearna Hartmann, for three months (from November 2014 to February 2015) to undertake some additional analysis of each edition of the *Diagnostic and Statistical Manual of Mental Disorders*. This work appears in Chaps. 3–7 of the book. Rearna should get a special mention here as she proved to be such an incredibly talented and efficient scholar-in-training; it was a real pleasure to work with you on this project.

For inspiration, support, and temporary escape from the book writing, I would like to thank my football team, Tripzville/University-Mt Wellington (the 2015 Division Three (Seniors) Over-35s champions!), especially the boss, Mark Rossi, and my left-back partner in the crime, Tony Westmoreland. The music from the Killers kept me reasonably buoyant throughout the writing phase. Thanks also to friends and family in England, Germany, Australia, and New Zealand for all the good times, including the constant flow of alcohol, much needed. Maeby and Milo constantly interrupted my writing to show me wildlife they had "found" in the garden; on reflection, probably useful exercise for me. Finally, from the east to the west, the north to the south, she is the love of my life and the brains of the operation, Dr Jessica Terruhn—thanks for all the feedback on the drafts and, you know, everything else. I love you, honey!

Contents

List of Abbreviations

ADD	Attention Deficit Disorder
ADHD	Attention-Deficit/Hyperactivity Disorder
APA	American Psychiatric Association*
APD	Antisocial Personality Disorder
BPD	Borderline Personality Disorder
CTO	Community Treatment Order
DSM	Diagnostic and Statistical Manual of Mental Disorders
ECT	Electroconvulsive Therapy
EL	Encephalitis Lethargica
FDA	Food and Drug Administration
GD	Gender Dysphoria
GID	Gender Identity Disorder
HPD	Histrionic Personality Disorder
ISA	Ideological State Apparatus
LLPDD	Late Luteal Phase Dysphoric Disorder
NIMH	National Institute of Mental Health
OSDD	Other Specified Dissociative Disorder
PENS	Psychological Ethics and National Security
PMDD	Premenstrual Dysphoric Disorder
PMS	Premenstrual Syndrome
PMT	Premenstrual Tension
PTSD	Posttraumatic Stress Disorder

SAD	Social Anxiety Disorder
SSRI	Selective Serotonin Reuptake Inhibitors
UK	United Kingdom
US	United States
WHO	World Health Organization
	(*to distinguish the American Psychiatric Association from the American Psychological Association, the full name for the latter is always given in the text)

List of Figures and Tables

1

Introduction: Thinking Critically About Mental Illness

This book is a critical reflection on the current global epidemic of mental disease, and with that, the global proliferation of mental health professionals and the expanding discourse on mental illness. Over the past 35 years, scientific ideas on mental pathology from the designated experts on the mind have seeped outwards from the psychiatric institution into many spheres of public and private life. It is part of my role as a sociologist to explain how this epidemic has come about and the extent to which it is a valid reflection of real medical progress in the area. I am not alone in undertaking such a project; other social scientists—as well as psychiatrists and psychologists themselves—have investigated the recent expansion in the varieties of mental disorder and their usage among western populations, and have voiced similar concerns to the ones that I will articulate in this book. However, as the title suggests, this work goes further than most other scholars and mental health experts appear able to. This is because I frame the business of mental health within its wider structural context, within a system of power relations of which economic exploitation is the determinant one. Ignoring the development and current dynamics of capitalist society has been a significant omission of most

B.M.Z. Cohen, *Psychiatric Hegemony*,
DOI 10.1057/978-1-137-46051-6_1

other scholarship in the area; this is my contribution to getting critical social theory back to the heart of research and scholarship in the sociology of mental health.

"We are," according to the psychotherapist James Davies (2013: 1), "a population on the brink." The figures for mental disease suggest that not only are we currently in the grip of an illness epidemic but we are nearing a tipping point towards catastrophe: out of a global population of seven billion inhabitants, 450 million people are estimated to be currently affected by a mental or behavioural disorder (World Health Organization 2003: 4), with 100 million of them taking psychotropic drugs (Chalasani 2016: 1184). The projected rates in developed countries such as the United States and the United Kingdom are even higher with one in four people suffering from a mental disorder each year (Davies 2013: 1). The World Health Organization (WHO) (2003: 5) estimates that the expenditure on mental health problems in western society amounts to between 3 and 4 per cent of gross national product; the cost in the United States alone is over $100 billion per year (Wilkinson and Pickett 2010: 65). By 2020, according to the WHO, depression—a disease which will affect one-fifth of all Americans at some point in their life (Horwitz and Wakefield 2007: 4)—will be "the second leading cause of worldwide disability, behind only heart disease" (Horwitz and Wakefield 2007: 5).

Consequently, the WHO (2003: 3) states of this mental illness epidemic that "[t]he magnitude, suffering and burden in terms of disability and costs for individuals, families and societies are staggering." From being a relatively rare affliction just 60 years ago, mental illness is now everybody's concern. Whitaker (2010a: 6–7) has noted of this change that the rates of debilitating mental illness among US adults has increased sixfold between 1955 and 2007. However, the "plague of disabling mental illness" as he calls it has fallen particularly hard on young people in the country, with an incredible *35-fold* increase between 1997 and 2007. This makes mental disease the "leading cause of disability in children" in the United States (Whitaker 2010a: 8). The varieties of known mental illnesses have also increased over time, with the American Psychiatric Association's (APA) *Diagnostic and Statistical*

Manual of Mental Disorders (DSM) identifying 106 mental disorders in 1952, yet 374 today (Davies 2013: 2).

In the current milieu it is no surprise that the power and influence of the mental health professionals are—like the above statistics—"growing at a remarkable rate" (Davies 2013: 2). However, as every critical scholar on the topic is aware, very serious problems remain with the current science and practice within the mental health system. These concerns inevitably lead us to questioning the reality of the claims to a mental illness "epidemic" made by health organisations such as the APA and the WHO, and to ask who really benefits from the global expansion of the psychiatric discourse. An essential issue here is the continuing contested nature of "mental illness," for there remains no proof that any "mental disorder" is a real, observable disease. Consequently, the "experts" still cannot distinguish the mentally ill from the mentally healthy. In fact, a recent attempt by the APA—the most powerful psychiatric body in the world—to define mental illness was bluntly described by one of their most senior figures as "bullshit" (see discussion below). Accordingly, it also follows that no "treatment" has been shown to work on any specific "mental illness" and that there is no known causation for any disorder. Of course, these issues are highly disputed by many mental health professionals, so the evidence and debates are outlined in detail in the chapters that follow.

I appreciate that questioning the validity of mental illness comes as little comfort to those people who are currently experiencing stress, trauma, or behaviour which causes what Thomas Szasz (1974) has previously referred to as "problems in living." Let me clarify briefly here that this book is not denying such experience; rather it is questioning the discourse of "mental illness" which is produced by groups of professionals who claim an expert knowledge over this experience. Therefore, the current discussion is a critique of professional power not of personal experience and behaviour which may have been labelled (or self-labelled) as a "mental illness." Though my previous work has investigated the multifaceted meanings of illness and recovery for those so labelled (see, e.g., Cohen 2015), this is not the focus of the current book. Instead, the issue at hand is how to explain the incredible expansion of what we might call the "mental health industry"—that is, the entirety of the professionals, businesses, and discourse surrounding the area of mental health and illness—without a concurrent progression in the scientific evidence on mental pathology. The next section briefly explores some of the main explanations given for the dominance of the current mental health system and the gaps in this work.

Critical Scholarship on Mental Illness

Most commonly, critical scholars focus on one major reason for the current expansion in the numbers and categories of mental illness in western society—namely, the influence of pharmaceutical corporations (colloquially referred to as "big pharma") on the construction of new categories of disorder and the promotion of drug solutions for those disorders (see, e.g., Davies 2013; Healy 2004; Moncrieff 2009; Moynihan and Cassels 2005; Whitaker 2010a; Whitaker and Cosgrove 2015). The institution of psychiatry is the ultimate authority responsible for defining and treating mental pathologies, yet commentators argue that the profession has been steadily compromised by forming close relationships with big pharma, who are now effectively setting the mental health agenda. For example, critics point to the 69 per cent of psychiatrists responsible for the development of the latest edition of the DSM (DSM-5, see American Psychiatric Association 2013) who have financial ties to the pharmaceutical industry (Cosgrove and Wheeler 2013: 95). Research has also demonstrated the close involvement of big pharma in the development of current mental illness categories including social anxiety disorder (SAD) (Lane 2007) and premenstrual dysphoric disorder (PMDD) (Cosgrove and Wheeler 2013). The more behaviour and experience that can be successfully medicalised—that is, reconceptualised as in need of medical intervention—through this medico-industrial partnership, the more drugs can be potentially sold to the public. Thus it is argued that the expansion of the mental illness discourse is the result of a market takeover of health care; corporations rather than medical practitioners are now designating what mental pathology is and, as a result, dictating treatment. The obvious solution to this situation involves the de-coupling of mental health services from the influence of big business. Tighter government regulation and oversight of pharmaceutical corporations is required, as is transparency within the relevant professional organisations.

While this critique of big pharma's intervention in the production and promotion of the contemporary psychiatric discourse is relevant, it is perhaps the least surprising aspect of the operation of the mental health system within capitalist society. Scholars of medical history such as Andrew Scull (1989, 1993, 2015), for example, have profiled a continuing "trade in lunacy" which can be traced back to the beginnings of industrial society and witnessed throughout the development of modern mental health work. That the market is part of the workings of psychiatry and related professions should be self-evident to any scholar aware of the history of the mental health system in western society. Such critics would also acknowledge that while psychiatry legitimates the products of big pharma, pushing psychopharmaceuticals in turn helps legitimate the psychiatric profession. The prescribing of drugs is a key symbol of modern doctoring which serves to align psychiatric practice with other branches of medicine through a shared biomedical understanding of health and illness.

The medico-industrial relationship described above has raised an associated criticism from critical scholars as to the efficacy of the biomedical approach in understanding mental health problems more generally. Biomedicine conceptualises disease as a physical pathology of the body. Thus, biomedical psychiatry theorises mental disorder as having a physical aetiology (causation) that can be observed, measured, and treated. Modern psychiatry focuses on the brain as the organ that causes such "disease," and most often regards mental illness as the result of faulty neurotransmitters or "chemical imbalances" in the brain. The biomedical approach to understanding mental illness have been a part of psychiatry since its emergence over 200 years ago, yet has become increasingly dominant within the mental health system since the 1980s (Chap. 2). According to critics, however, despite its current "hegemonic" moment (Cosgrove and Wheeler 2013: 100), bio-psychiatry lacks the legitimacy of scientific evidence. The scholars blame corrupt individuals and powerful interests both inside and outside of psychiatry for reiterating biomedical myths regarding the "normal" and "abnormal" workings of the brain so as to be able to promote physical interventions such as drugs and electroconvulsive therapy (ECT) as potential "cures" for mental illness. Such writers note the continuing lack of proof of biological causation for any mental disorder, the potential for corruption at the hands of big pharma, the perversion of the psychiatric profession by particular self-interested, powerful parties and individuals, and the reductionist nature of the biomedical model which is seen to have damaged the founding aims of the profession to improve the care and treatment of people who suffer from mental disorders and to always perform their duties in the best interests of the patient (see, e.g., Bentall 2009; Breggin 1991; Davies 2013; Greenberg 2013; Whitaker and Cosgrove 2015).

Critics call for an understanding of mental disorder which goes beyond biological reductionism to consider psychological, social, and environmental factors which correlate with mental illness. Often conceptualised as the "psychosocial model" (or simply, the "social model") of mental illness, scholars and experts highlight a range of evidence from socio-economic data which demonstrates that such factors as family income, educational level, ethnic group, geographical location, and social class are all closely related to the chances of developing a mental health problem. While the social model suggests that we all have the potential to suffer mental disorders if exposed to traumatic situations, some groups are particularly vulnerable to mental illness due to experiencing comparatively more stressful life conditions and, at the same time, having less access to cultural and economic resources which can alleviate the threat of mental problems. As the WHO's (2013) recent *Mental Health Action Plan 2013–2020* has emphasised,

> Depending on the local context, certain individuals and groups in society may be placed at a significantly higher risk of experiencing mental health problems. These vulnerable groups may (but do not necessarily) include members of households living in poverty, people with chronic health conditions, infants and children exposed to maltreatment and neglect, adolescents first exposed to substance use, minority groups, indigenous populations, older people, people experiencing discrimination and human rights violations, lesbian, gay, bisexual, and transgender persons, prisoners, and people exposed to conflict, natural disasters or other humanitarian emergencies.

Interventions are then aimed at the personal and the social; therapy and counselling allows individuals to work through their disorder with trained professionals, while community health services target certain deprived communities for mental health promotions and the additional resourcing of mental illness prevention teams.

Explanations for the increase in rates of mental illness given by socially orientated models of mental health, therefore, draw attention to the widening social inequalities experienced in neoliberal society which impact levels of well-being in vulnerable populations. For example, Wilkinson and Pickett (2010: 67) draw on WHO data to claim that people suffer more mental illness in countries with wider inequalities (as measured by income distribution and the disparities between the richest and the poorest in that society). Their comparison of twelve advanced industrial nations shows the United States as having the highest rates of mental illness and, correspondingly, the highest rate of income inequalities. In comparison, Japan experiences the lowest rate of mental health problems and has a relatively equal distribution of income. It is a popular piece of sociologically orientated accounting in which society has the potential to make us sick; particularly those societies with higher levels of social and economic inequality appear to make us sicker. Thus, some Marxists have similarly argued that capitalism is ultimately responsible for causing mental illness (see, e.g., Robinson 1997; Rosenthal and Campbell 2016). However, as with most epidemiological work on mental illness, this analysis is weak and inconclusive. The research ultimately suffers from the same fundamental deficit as the biomedical model in that, while speculative correlations are made, there remains no proof of causation for any mental disorder.

As with psychiatrists, the many mental health workers in allied professions—such as the psychotherapists, psychologists, counsellors, and psychiatric social workers—who promote the more socially orientated approaches to mental illness, continue to stand by the validity of psychiatry's knowledge base and for good reason: it is a discourse which furthers their own professional interests and legitimates their own "mental health" practices in a currently expanding market. Many scholars make the same mistake in arguing for such socially oriented approaches—they reinforce the psychiatric discourse as having validity where none has been established. Thus, what may first appear as serious critical scholarship on psychiatric knowledge production and the mental health system is often quite conservative and reformist in nature. These attempts at "critical" literature on the mental health system are most likely written by those inside the mental health profession, especially psychiatrists and psychologists (see, e.g., Bentall 2009; Davies 2013; Paris 2008). Unless they wish to give up their high-paid jobs—some escape into academia, others retire early—these writers continue to be complicit in supporting the mental health system that has produced them. For this reason their arguments go no further than pleas for reform (fewer drugs, more therapy, and so on) which allow their profession to continue to expand their operations relatively unhindered by serious critique.

To firmly ground the mental health system as a moral and political project, the following section discusses the continuing lack of validity of psychiatric knowledge. This deconstruction of the "science" of psychiatry is purposely undertaken here to highlight both the limits of previous critical scholarship—which has often failed to engage with the fundamental problems of mental health work—and the need to frame such institutions within structural systems of power and social control. Before this however, a brief note on a couple of key terms I will use in this discussion and subsequently throughout the book.

Psy-professions: my argument in this book implicates not only the psychiatric profession, but also allied groups such as psychologists, counsellors, psychiatric social workers, psychoanalysts, and the many other "talk therapy" professionals (for full critiques, see, e.g., Masson 1994; Morrall 2008). Collectively, I follow Rose (1999: viii) in understanding these groups as the "psy-professions": "experts" who have over time acquired an authority on the supposed "real nature of humans as psychological subjects." As medically trained practitioners, psychiatrists have the ultimate authority to define and police abnormal behaviour—which is why the book focuses primarily on this profession—yet they are ably assisted by other groups which have subsequently emerged and have vested interests in continuing to align themselves with the same knowledge base. The discussion in this book will demonstrate, for example, that psychologists, therapists, and counsellors can all be implicated in systematically serving the interests of the powerful.

Psychiatric discourse: I use this term to differentiate scientific evidence on "mental illness" (what some might call "psychiatric knowledge," although this is also a highly problematic phrase) from psy-professional claims-making in the area. Psychiatric discourse is the totality of the propositions to expertise on "mental illness" and "mental health" (including the language, practices, and treatments) that psychiatric and allied professions have circulated to the public over the past 200 years. The term signifies the socially constructed nature of what is claimed to be expert knowledge in the area. For this reason, general terminology produced by the mental health system should be treated with caution. For example, in this book I refer to various labels of "mental illness," to mental health "experts," to "patients" and "users" of services, and so on; this does not, however, signal my acceptance of any such terminology as accurate or the truth of the matter.

Deconstructing the "Science" of Psychiatry

In his recent book *Shrinks: The Untold Story of Psychiatry*, former president of the APA, Jeffrey Lieberman (2015: 288–289), summarises the progress that psychiatry has made over the past 200 years in its knowledge and understanding of mental pathology. "We know that mental disorders exhibit consistent clusters of symptoms," he declares,

> We know that many disorders feature distinctive neural signatures in the brain. We know that many disorders express distinctive patterns of brain activity. We have gained some insight into the genetic underpinnings of mental disorders. We can treat persons with mental disorders using medications and somatic therapies that act uniquely on their symptoms but exert no effects in healthy people. We know that specific types of psychotherapy lead to clear improvements in patients suffering from specific types of disorders. And we know that, left untreated, these disorders cause anguish, misery, disability, violence, even death. Thus, mental disorders are abnormal, enduring, harmful, treatable, feature a biological component, and can be reliably diagnosed.

Underscoring psychiatry's worth as a medical enterprise, Lieberman (2015: 289) concludes by stating of the above summary that "I believe this should satisfy anyone's definition of medical illness." Likewise, Shorter (1997: 325) concurs with Lieberman on the ascendancy of the psychiatric discipline to a valid branch of medical science when he reflects that

> [i]n two hundred years ... psychiatrists [have] progressed from being the healers of the therapeutic asylum to serving as gatekeepers for Prozac. Psychiatric illness has passed from a feared sign of bad blood—a genetic curse—to an easily treatable condition not essentially different from any other medical problem, and possessing roughly the same affective valence.

Such positive appraisal of the knowledge and treatment of mental disorders by the official historians of psychiatry necessarily rationalises the jurisdictional exclusivity of the profession as based on a progressive narrative of medical science and discovery. Nevertheless, it is a successfully cultivated rhetoric of truth claims which crucially lacks evidence to sustain the desired picture of medical advancement in the field. This section surveys the main issues with the current state of psychiatric knowledge—namely, the disagreements over aetiology and treatment of mental illness, the lack of agreement on what "mental illness" is, and consequently the lack of validity to any category of mental disorder. This deconstruction of psychiatric knowledge claims will lead us to question what the purpose of the psy-professions in capitalist society actually is.

A recent review of the science behind the psychiatric discourse concluded that "no biological sign has ever been found for any 'mental disorder.' Correspondingly, there is no known physiological etiology" (Burstow 2015: 75). This conclusion also became clear to the APA's own DSM-5 task force when they began work on the new manual in 2002. As Whitaker and Cosgrove (2015: 60) record, in reviewing the available research evidence it was plain to the committee members that "[t]he etiology of mental disorders remained unknown. The field [of mental health] still did not have a biological marker or genetic test that could be used for diagnostic purposes." Furthermore, the research also showed that psychiatrists could still not distinguish between mentally healthy and mentally sick people, and consequently had failed to define their area of supposed expertise. This issue was recently highlighted with reference to comments made by Allen Frances, the chair of the previous DSM-IV task force. When the DSM-IV (American Psychiatric Association 1994: xxi) was published in 1994, it stated that "mental disorder" was

> conceptualized as a clinically significant behavioral or psychological syndrome or pattern that occurs in an individual and that is associated with

> present distress (e.g., a painful symptom) or disability (i.e., impairment in one or more important areas of functioning) or with a significantly increased risk of suffering death, pain, disability, or an important loss of freedom.

However, as the architect of the DSM-IV, Frances was later quoted by Greenberg (2013: 35–36) as stating of the above definition, "[h]ere's the problem … There is no definition of a mental disorder … it's bullshit … I mean you can't define it." The lack of knowledge on mental health and illness has haunted the entire history of psychiatry. Some have dismissed critics who highlight this fundamental hole in the science of psychiatry as "antipsychiatry" or "mental illness deniers." Such attacks on scholars who attempt to investigate the accuracy of the central pillars of psychiatric knowledge should further concern us, as it perhaps signals that plenty in the profession are already aware of the flimsy nature on which their "expertise" continues to rest. Together with an understanding of the history of the psychiatric profession—summed up by Scull (1989: 8) as "dismal and depressing"—I would argue that it should be the duty of *all* social scientists concerned with the mental health field that, in good conscience and putting the needs of the public first, they remain highly sceptical of a psychiatric discourse that poses as expert knowledge on the mind but produces little actual evidence to back up the assertions made.

Though at first glance historical mental disorders such as masturbatory insanity (Chap. 2), drapetomania (Chap. 7), hysteria (Chap. 5), and homosexuality may appear as evidence of the profession reflecting the dominant norms and values of wider society, they are argued by the official historians of psychiatry to be examples of the false starts, early experimentations, and theoretical innovations of an emerging scientific discipline. It is suggested that this history is evidence of medical and scientific progress within the area of mental health to the current point where we know more about mental distress than ever before. Yet problems in the legitimacy of psychiatry's vocation have remained, and reached crisis point at the cusp of deinstitutionalisation in the 1970s. At the time, a number of significant studies demonstrated the profession's inherent tendency to label people as "mentally ill," to stigmatise everyday aspects of a person's behaviour as signs of pathology, and to make judgements on a person's mental health status based on subjective judgements rather than objective criteria.

The study that had the most direct impact on the psychiatric profession—as well as public consciousness—at this time was David Rosenhan's (1973) classic research *On Being Sane in Insane Places* which found that psychiatrists could not distinguish between "real" and "pseudo" patients presenting at psychiatric hospitals in the United States. All of Rosenhan's "pseudo" patients (college students/researchers involved in the experiment) were admitted and given a psychotic label, and all the subsequent behaviour of the researchers—including their note-taking—was labelled by staff as further symptoms of their disorder (for a summary, see Burstow 2015: 75–76). This research was a culmination of earlier studies on labelling and mental illness which had begun in the 1960s with Irving Goffman (1961) and Thomas Scheff (1966). Goffman's (1961) ethnographic study of psychiatric incarceration demonstrated many of the features which Rosenhan's study would later succinctly outline, including the arbitrary nature of psychiatric assessment, the labelling of patient behaviour as further evidence of "mental illness," and the processes of institutional conformity by which the inmates learned to accept such labels if they wanted to have any chance of being released from the institution at a later date. Scheff's (1966) work on diagnostic decision making in psychiatry formulated a general labelling theory for the sociology of mental health. Again, his research found that psychiatrists made arbitrary and subjective decisions on those designated as "mentally ill," sometimes retaining people in institutions even when there was no evidence to support such a decision. Psychiatrists, he argued, relied on a common sense set of beliefs and practices rather than observable, scientific evidence. Scheff (1966) concluded that the labelling of a person with a "mental illness" was contingent on the violation of social norms by low-status rule-breakers who are judged by higher status agents of social control (in this case, the psychiatric profession). Thus, according to these studies, the nature of "mental illness" is not a fixed object of medical study but rather a form of "social deviance"—a moral marker of societal infraction by the powerful inflicted on the powerless. This situation is summated in Becker's (1963: 9, emphasis original) general theory of social deviance which stated that

> deviance is *not* a quality of the act the person commits, but rather a consequence of the application by others of rules and sanctions to an "offender." The deviant is one to whom that label has successfully been applied; deviant behavior is behavior that people so label.

The growing perception that psychiatric work was "unscientific" and, in turn, "mental illness" was a label of social deviance was further amplified in the 1970s by the APA's very public battle over the continuation of homosexuality as a classification of mental disorder in the DSM (for a full discussion, see Kutchins and Kirk 1997: 55–99). As with the rationale for the profession labelling this sexual orientation as a mental illness in both the DSM-I (American Psychiatric Association 1952: 38–39) and the DSM-II (American Psychiatric Association 1968: 44), the successful decision to subsequently remove the label from the manual in 1973 was anything but scientific. On the contrary, Burstow (2015: 80) records how a mix of disruptive protests by gay rights campaigners, along with an internal power struggle between psychoanalysts and biomedical-orientated psychiatrists, brought about the change in APA policy. The end result was a decision based not on research evidence but rather a simple postal vote of APA members (Burstow 2015: 80). With institutional psychiatry in decline, community alternatives developing, and related mental health disciplines encroaching on traditional psychiatric territory, the profession entered a period of political and epistemological crisis. To regain credibility, the APA needed to prove the robustness of its knowledge base and convince the public as well as policy makers of their continuing usefulness and expertise.

The solution was to boost the scientific credibility of the field through improving the reliability of mental illness categories—that is, the identification and agreement among different practitioners of patients presenting with a specific disorder—which would then aid in validating such pathologies as real disease rather than professionally produced constructions. As Whitaker and Cosgrove (2015: 45–46) state of the importance of the reliability and validity concepts,

> In infectious medicine, a diagnostic manual needs to be both reliable and valid in order to be truly useful. A classification system that is reliable enables physicians to distinguish between different diseases, and to then prescribe a treatment specific to a disease, which has been validated—through studies of its clinical course and, if possible, an understanding of its pathology—as real.

Under the leadership of Robert Spitzer, the APA carried out extensive field trials with the aim of testing the reliability of different diagnostic categories towards the creation of a more robust and scientifically sound DSM (to be released in 1980 as the DSM-III). Spitzer and Fleiss' (cited in Kirk and Kutchins 1994: 75) own assessment of the reliability of categories of mental disorder in the DSM-I and the DSM-II was that none of them were more than "satisfactory," frankly admitting that

> [t]here are no diagnostic categories for which reliability is uniformly high. Reliability appears only satisfactory for three categories: mental deficiency, organic brain syndrome (but not its subtypes), and alcoholism. The level of reliability is no better than fair for psychosis and schizophrenia and is poor for the remaining categories.

To rectify this situation, Spitzer's team coordinated a number of large-scale pieces of research on psychiatric classification, including "the largest reliability study in history" (Burstow 2015: 77; for full details, see Williams et al. 1992) involving 592 people—both psychiatric patients and those without a previous history of mental health problems—being interviewed by pairs of psychiatrists spread over six sites in the United States and one in Germany. Kirk and Kutchins (1994: 83) have described the time, planning, and resourcing that went into this study as "the envy of researchers who attempt to conduct rigorous studies in clinical settings." Subsequently, the data was claimed by the developers of the DSM-III to be of "far greater reliability" for most classes of mental disorder than that utilised in previous DSMs; the results showed a generally "quite good" level of agreement between psychiatrists, especially on the classic categories of schizophrenia and major affective disorders (American Psychiatric Association, cited in Kirk and Kutchins 1994: 79). On its release in 1980, the DSM-III was hailed as a great success for the discipline—a document which would finally silence detractors through accurately demonstrating the effective scientific progress of the discipline in the twentieth century. Consequently, the DSM-III has come to mark a "revolution" within the discipline (Decker 2013: xv). For western psychiatry, the manual was the "book that changed everything" (Lieberman 2015: 134).

It was, however, a revolution based on a scientific lie. The DSM-III field trials were "[b]latently rigged" (Burstow 2015: 77) by Spitzer's task force to produce higher rates of reliability. A summary of the research biases in the construction of the studies—including the non-representative nature of the samples—has been noted by Whitaker and Cosgrove (2015: 48–49), following extensive meta-analysis of the original field trial data by Kirk and Kutchins (1992). However, Kirk and Kutchins' own evaluation of the DSM-III research revealed something even more surprising—namely, that there was no improvement in the previous poor levels of diagnostic reliability. In fact, in some categories of mental disorder, there were even *greater levels of disagreement* between psychiatrists than there had been with previous DSMs (Kirk and Kutchins 1994: 82–83). In large part, the claimed success of the DSM-III was due to a "linguistic sleight of hand" (Whitaker and Cosgrove 2015: 49) in which Spitzer and his task force re-phrased the same statistical levels of agreement between psychiatric professions (in this case, defined by kappa mean values between 0 and 1, where 1 is complete agreement and 0 complete disagreement) in different ways when comparing the DSM-I and the DSM-II with the DSM-III. For example, a mental disorder in the previous DSMs with a kappa score of .7 had been presented as "only satisfactory," but was then redefined in the DSM-III as a "good" level of inter-rater agreement (Whitaker and Cosgrove 2015: 49). Thus, Kirk and Kutchins (1994: 83) concluded that "despite the scientific claims of great success, reliability appears to have improved very little in three decades." The DSM-III can therefore be seen as the success of the rhetoric of psychiatry rather than the result of any actual scientific progress within the discipline (Kirk and Kutchins 1992).

Predictably, subsequent research has shown no improvement in inter-rater reliability and, in many cases, has produced kappa scores below those reported in the original DSM-III field trials (Whitaker and Cosgrove 2015: 50). The implications for the DSM on which psychiatry bases its claims to scientific rigour are clear—"the latest versions of DSM as a clinical tool," state Kirk and Kutchins (1994: 84), "are unreliable and therefore of questionable validity as a classification system." As the authors proceeded to document with the DSM-IV, rather than attempt to tighten mental illness classifications, the APA actually loosened them further, thereby increasing the potential number of people who could be labelled under each mental disorder (Kutchins and Kirk 1997). Following the DSM-III field trials, subsequent DSM task forces have abandoned the reliability issue, believing it to have been solved despite ongoing criticisms from health researchers and social scientists. And, lest we forget, even if psychiatry did one day solve the reliability problem, it still does not solve the validity issue for mental disorder classifications. After all, "[t]he fact that people can be trained to apply a label in a consistent way," Burstow (2015: 78) reminds us, "does not mean that the label points to anything real."

Psychiatric insiders have openly admitted the lack of science to their area of operations. Allen Frances (cited in Whitaker and Cosgrove 2015: 61), for example, has recently stated that the mental disorders given in the DSM are "better understood as no more than currently convenient constructs or heuristics that allow [psychiatrists] to communicate with one another." This has included the classic constructs of schizophrenia and bipolar disorder (formerly manic-depression), of which the mental health researcher Joel Paris at the Department of Psychiatry, McGill University, has admitted "[i]n reality, we do not know whether [such] conditions ... are true diseases" (cited in Whitaker and Cosgrove 2015: 61). Even National Institute of Mental Health (NIMH) director and strong advocate of biomedical psychiatry, Thomas Insel (cited in Masson 2015: xii), announced on the release of the DSM-5 in 2013 that the categories of mental disorder lacked validity and NIMH would no longer be using such diagnoses for research purposes.

Despite the claims to "progress" made by official historians of psychiatry such as Lieberman and Shorter, there is no evidence for the supposed "science" of psychiatry. There is no test for any mental illness, no proof of causation, no evidence of successful "treatment" that relates specifically to an individual disorder, and no accurate prediction of future cases. Thus, the claim that psychiatric constructs are real disease has not been proven. Consequently, it is necessary to utilise the existing evidence to more accurately theorise the real vocation of the psy-professions in capitalist society. As the faulty knowledge claims of the DSM are summarised by Burstow (2015: 78, emphasis original), "reliability cannot legitimately function as a validity claim and no studies have established validity"; therefore, "it follows that ... no foundation *of any sort* exists for the DSM categories. This is a serious issue that calls into question the power vested in psychiatry." It necessarily leads us to consider such institutions as moral and political enterprises rather than medical ones (Szasz 1974: xii) because psy-professionals make historically and culturally bound judgements on the "correct" and "appropriate" behaviour of society's members. This is a point summated by Ingelby (1980: 55, emphasis added) when he states that

> what one thinks psychiatrists are up to depends crucially on what one thinks their patients are up to; and *the latter question cannot be answered without taking an essentially political stand on what constitutes a "reasonable" response to a social situation.*

In the same manner, British psychiatrist Joanna Moncrieff (2010: 371) agrees that a "psychiatric diagnosis can be understood as functioning as a political device, in the sense that it legitimates a particular social response to aberrant behaviour of various sorts, but protects that response from any democratic challenge." Even Shorter (1997: viii) accepts that the profession is responsible for policing social deviance when he remarks that "[p]sychiatry is, to be sure, the ultimate rulemaker of acceptable behaviour through its ability to specify what counts as 'crazy.'" Likewise, the concept of "health" within the mental health system is understood as whatever counts as "normal" within a specific historical epoch and cultural setting. Sayers (cited in Christian 1997: 33–34) states of this relative concept of "health" that

> [t]he society and the individual's role within it are assumed to be normal (that is to say, "healthy": "normality" is a common synonym for "health" in psychiatry as in other areas of medicine). Indeed, the prevailing social environment is made the very criterion of normality, and the individual is judged ill insofar as he or she fails to "adjust" to it.

The Urgency for Marxist Theory

Despite the lack of validity to the "science" of psychiatry, most "critical" texts fail to adequately explain the expansion of mental health work because they lack sustained *theoretical engagement*. Most commentators refuse to conceptualise the mental health business beyond what they can see with their own eyes, and this in turn hides the wider structural forces which can shape, inhabit, and direct the institutional priorities of the mental health experts. For instance, if Wilkinson and Pickett (2010: 67) had spent more time critically investigating the production of psychiatric knowledge, they might have come to the conclusion that the more unequal the society, the more likely it is that people will be *labelled* with a mental disorder. Stated in a slightly different manner, countries that have faced the brunt of neoliberal polices are more likely to apply labels of "mental disorder" onto the population.

This is not, however, to suggest that there has been a complete absence of critical social theorising on the activities of the psy-professionals within capitalist society. On the contrary, from labelling and social constructionist accounts to critical realism, post-psychiatry, and mad studies, there has been a considerable tradition of engagement with the issues of societal inequalities, institutional power, and psychiatric mechanisms of social control since the 1960s (see Cohen, forthcoming). Such literature has been highly valuable to the sociology of mental health and is utilised throughout this book. Nevertheless, this scholarship still fails to fully contextualise the political project of psychiatry in relation to the fundamental conditions of economic exploitation under capitalism. The critical analysis lacks either a full understanding of the dynamics of capitalist society or an adequate historical and contemporary contextualisation of the institution of psychiatry. Without attending to both of these issues, the scholarship will remain piecemeal and theoretically incomplete. It is my contention that an inherently political institution such as psychiatry can only be fully understood through an appropriate framing of the profession within wider socio-historical processes and with the aid of Marxist theory. This allows us to make sense of the emergence and development of the psy-professions within industrial society, their changing practices and priorities, points of internal and external competition and conflict, as well as their current period of expansion in neoliberal society.

It has been left to a small handful of Marxist scholars to outline a fundamental truth of the mental health system: that its priorities and practices are fundamentally shaped by the goals of capitalism (see, e.g., Brown 1974; Nahem 1981; Parker 2007; Roberts 2015; Robinson 1997; Rosenthal and Campbell 2016). As Brown (1974: 1) has remarked of psychology, it is "more than just a professional field of work. It is also a codified ideology and practice that arises from the nature of our capitalist society and functions to bolster that society." This is less surprising, states Nahem (1981: 7), when it is understood that, as with psychiatry, "[p]sychology arose and developed in capitalist society, a class society. In all class societies, the dominant social, cultural and political views are those of the dominant class." And more so, with the continuing expansion of the psy-professions, Parker (2007: 1–2) argues that psychology has become

> an increasingly powerful component of ideology, ruling ideas that endorse exploitation and sabotage struggles against oppression. This psychology circulates way beyond colleges and clinics, and different versions of psychology as ideology are now to be found nearly everywhere in capitalist society.

The dominant norms and values of the ruling classes are reflected in the psychiatric discourse on human behaviour and the workings of the mind. Consequently, the psy-professions are responsible for facilitating the maximisation of profit for the ruling classes while individualising the social and economic conditions of the workers. The mental health system seeks to normalise the fundamentally oppressive relations of capitalism by focusing on the individual—rather than the society—as pathological and in need of adjustment through "treatment" options such as drugs, ECT, and therapy. These arguments will be discussed in further detail in the chapters that follow. To end this section, however, I briefly want to highlight a key problem with previous Marxist literature.

Almost all of the Marxist scholars cited above come from inside the psy-professions (usually psychology), and for that reason most attempt to still rescue their discipline from capitalism. For example, Nahem (1981: 7) speaks of the mental health system as being "co-opted" by capitalism, a situation in which the true evidence-based practice of psychiatry and psychology has been replaced by the ideology of the ruling classes. Similarly, Robinson (1997) and Rosenthal and Campbell (2016) argue that the psy-professions have been tainted by capitalism, and that, consequently, a socialist society would have "a genuinely scientific psychology [which] will constitute an essential part of human culture" (Robinson 1997: 77). However, the idea of a "new psychiatry" or "new psychology" based on Marxist principles (as suggested in Brown 1974) is fundamentally incompatible with the socio-historical reality of these institutions (Chap. 2). As I argue throughout this book, the psy-professions are a product of capitalism; they were created to police dissent and reinforce conformity, not to emancipate people. Thus, they cannot be reformed or rescued from capitalism; they are and will always be institutions of social control, and for that reason they have no positive role to play in a socialist society (Chap. 8). As important as the previous Marxist scholarship on mental health has been, this book avoids the potential biases of the reformed therapist, psychologist, or psychiatrist in assessing the history and current expansion of the psy-professionals.

Summary

Twenty years ago, Thomas Harris (1995: xv), the bestselling author of *I'm OK-You're OK*—one of the first "popular psychology" texts on the market—stated that "[t]he question [for psychiatry] has always been how to get Freud off the couch and to the masses." This book explains how and why the psychiatric discourse has proliferated over the past few decades and achieved its current hegemonic status in neoliberal society. The following chapter appropriately grounds the discussion in Marx's classic theory of historical materialism. This is contextualised within a socio-historical analysis of the philosophies and treatments of the psychiatric profession over the past 200 years. The discussion demonstrates how the mental health system has served both the economic and ideological needs of capitalist society. With reference to the work of neo-Marxist scholarship, the specific linkage of neoliberalism to the expansion of the psychiatric discourse is explained in Chap. 3. The "crisis" of psychiatry in the mid-1970s and the construction of the DSM-III in 1980 need to be understood within the wider political framework of a declining welfare state and an increasing focus on individualism. To explore how the psy-professionals serve capitalist society in specific areas of private and public life, Chaps. 4–7 analyse the impingement of psychiatric hegemony on young people and women, as well as in work lives and with forms of social and political protest. Each of these chapters includes textual research on the DSM, demonstrating how categories and symptoms of mental disorder have come to increasingly mirror the dominant norms and values of neoliberal society. Chapter 4 investigates the psychological sciences' engagement with the world of work, including a case study of social anxiety disorder—the construction of which can only be fully understood in the context of neoliberal demands for "employability" and "sellable selves" within the labour force. As part of the future workforce, Chap. 5 investigates the growth in mental disorders aimed specifically at young people. Including a socio-historical analysis of the most commonly diagnosed childhood mental illness (attention-deficit/hyperactivity disorder (ADHD)), the discussion demonstrates that the contemporary moment of labelling children with mental disorders is strongly related to the requirements of late capitalism for compliant, disciplined, and higher-skilled workers. In comparison to the mental health system's relatively recent focus on young people, women have been an ongoing obsession for the psy-professions since the beginning of industrial society. From hysteria to borderline personality disorder (BPD), Chap. 6 recounts the systematic pathologisation of female emotions and experiences by psy-professionals, showing how these activities have primarily functioned to reinforce the division of labour, traditional gender roles, and patriarchal power. Chapter 7 explores some of the darkest moments in the history of the mental health system including their support for slavery, the central role they played in the Nazi holocaust, and their recent involvement in torturing prisoners of the "war on terror." This discussion will demonstrate that, rather than being isolated events carried out by rogue elements, these activities achieved widespread support among the mental health experts and were fundamentally considered to be "in the best interests of the patient." Further, the analysis will also show that the post-9/11 "culture of fear" in western society has only served to further enforce psychiatry hegemony, a situation achieved through the closer surveillance of social and political dissent as reflected in the DSM-5. Chapter 8 concludes the discussion in this book by briefly offering a few practical ways in which we can begin to challenge the psychiatric hegemon. These include challenging the academic apologists for the psy-professions, campaigning for the outlawing of psychiatric violence and compulsory treatment, and the forming of alliances with fellow radical scholars, psychiatric survivors, and left-wing activists.

Bibliography

American Psychiatric Association. (1952) *Diagnostic and Statistical Manual: Mental Disorders*. Washington, DC: American Psychiatric Association.

American Psychiatric Association. (1968) *Diagnostic and Statistical Manual of Mental Disorders* (2nd ed.). Washington, DC: American Psychiatric Association.

American Psychiatric Association. (1994) *Diagnostic and Statistical Manual of Mental Disorders* (4th ed.). Washington, DC: American Psychiatric Association.

American Psychiatric Association. (2013) *Diagnostic and Statistical Manual of Mental Disorders* (5th ed.). Arlington, VA: American Psychiatric Association.

Becker, H. S. (1963) *Outsiders: Studies in the Sociology of Deviance*. New York: The Free Press.

Bentall, R. P. (2009) *Doctoring The Mind: Why Psychiatric Treatments Fail*. London: Penguin.

Breggin, P. R. (1991) *Toxic Psychiatry: Why Therapy, Empathy, and Love Must Replace the Drugs, Electroshock, and Biochemical Theories of the 'New Psychiatry'*. New York: St. Martin's Press.

Brown, P. (1974) *Towards a Marxist Psychology*. New York: Harper & Row.

Burstow, B. (2015) *Psychiatry and the Business of Madness: An Ethical and Epistemological Accounting*. New York: Palgrave Macmillan.

Chalasani, P. (2016) 'Psychopharmacology', in Boslaugh, S. E. (Ed.), *The Sage Encyclopedia of Pharmacology and Society* (pp. 1180–1190). Thousand Oaks: Sage.

Christian, J. M. (1997) 'The Body as a Site of Reproduction and Resistance: Attention Deficit Hyperactivity Disorder and the Classroom', *Interchange*, 28(1): 31–43.

Cohen, B. M. Z. (2015) *Mental Health User Narratives: New Perspectives on Illness and Recovery* (rev. ed.). Houndmills, Basingstoke: Palgrave Macmillan.

Cohen, B. M. Z. (ed.) (forthcoming) *Routledge International Handbook of Critical Mental Health*. Abingdon: Routledge.

Cosgrove, L., and Wheeler, E. E. (2013) 'Industry's Colonization of Psychiatry: Ethical and Practical Implications of Financial Conflicts of Interest in the DSM-5', *Feminism & Psychology*, 23(1): 93–106.

Davies, J. (2013) *Cracked: Why Psychiatry is Doing More Harm than Good.* London: Icon Books.
Decker, H. S. (2013) *The Making of DSM-III: A Diagnostic Manual's Conquest of American Psychiatry.* Oxford: Oxford University Press.
Goffman, E. (1961) *Asylums: Essays on the Social Situation of Mental Patients and Other Inmates.* London: Penguin.
Greenberg, G. (2013) *The Book of Woe: The DSM and The Unmaking of Psychiatry.* New York: Blue Rider Press.
Harris, T. A. (1995) *I'm OK-You're OK.* London: Arrow Books.
Healy, D. (2004) *Let Them Eat Prozac: The Unhealthy Relationship Between the Pharmaceutical Industry and Depression.* New York: New York University Press.
Horwitz, A. V., and Wakefield, J. C. (2007) *The Loss of Sadness: How Psychiatry Transformed Normal Sorrow into Depressive Disorder.* New York: Oxford University Press.
Ingelby, D. (1980) 'Understanding "Mental Illness"', in Ingelby, D. (Ed.), *Critical Psychiatry: The Politics of Mental Health* (pp. 23–71). New York: Pantheon Books.
Kirk, S. A., and Kutchins, H. (1992) *The Selling of DSM: The Rhetoric of Science in Psychiatry.* New York: Aldine De Gruyter.
Kirk, S. A., and Kutchins, H. (1994) 'The Myth of the Reliability of DSM', *Journal of Mind and Behavior,* 15(1/2): 71–86.
Kutchins, H., and Kirk, S. A. (1997) *Making Us Crazy: DSM: The Psychiatric Bible and the Creation of Mental Disorders.* New York: Free Press.
Lane, C. (2007) *Shyness: How Normal Behavior Became a Sickness.* New Haven: Yale University Press.
Lieberman, J. A. (2015) *Shrinks: The Untold Story of Psychiatry.* New York: Little, Brown and Company.
Masson, J. M. (1994) *Against Therapy* (rev. ed.). Monroe: Common Courage Press.
Masson, J. M. (2015) 'Forward', in Cohen, B. M. Z. (Ed.), *Mental Health User Narratives: New Perspectives on Illness and Recovery* (rev. ed.). Houndmills, Basingstoke: Palgrave Macmillan.
Moncrieff, J. (2009) *The Myth of Chemical Cure: A Critique of Psychiatric Drug Treatment* (rev. ed.). Houndmills, Basingstoke: Palgrave Macmillan.
Moncrieff, J. (2010) 'Psychiatric Diagnosis as a Political Device', *Social Theory & Health,* 8(4): 370–382.
Morrall, P. (2008) *The Trouble with Therapy: Sociology and Psychotherapy.* Maidenhead: McGraw Hill/Open University Press.

Moynihan, R., and Cassels, A. (2005) *Selling Sickness: How Drug Companies are Turning Us All into Patients*. Crows Nest: Allen and Unwin.
Nahem, J. (1981) *Psychology and Psychiatry Today: A Marxist View*. New York: International Publishers.
Paris, J. (2008) *Prescriptions for the Mind: A Critical View of Contemporary Psychiatry*. Oxford: Oxford University Press.
Parker, I. (2007) *Revolution in Psychology: Alienation to Emancipation*. London: Pluto Press.
Roberts, R. (2015) *Psychology and Capitalism: The Manipulation of Mind*. Alresford: Zero Books.
Robinson, J. (1997) *The Failure of Psychiatry: A Marxist Critique*. London: Index Books.
Rose, N. (1999) *Governing the Soul: The Shaping of the Private Self* (2nd ed.). London: Free Association Books.
Rosenhan, D. L. (1973) 'On Being Sane in Insane Places', *Science*, 179(4070): 250–258.
Rosenthal, S., and Campbell, P. (2016) *Marxism and Psychology*. Toronto: ReMarx Publishing.
Scheff, T. J. (1966) *Being Mentally Ill: A Sociological Theory*. Chicago: Aldine.
Scull, A. (1989) *Social Order/Mental Disorder: Anglo-American Psychiatry in Historical Perspective*. Berkeley: University of California Press.
Scull, A. (1993) *The Most Solitary of Afflictions: Madness and Society in Britain, 1700–1900*. New Haven: Yale University Press.
Scull, A. (2015) *Madness in Civilization: A Cultural History of Insanity, from the Bible to Freud, from the Madhouse to Modern Medicine*. Princeton: Princeton University Press.
Shorter, E. (1997) *A History of Psychiatry: From the Era of the Asylum to the Age of Prozac*. New York: John Wiley & Sons.
Szasz, T. S. (1974) *The Myth of Mental Illness: Foundations of a Theory of Personal Conduct* (rev. ed.). New York: Harper & Row.
Whitaker, R. (2010a) *Anatomy of an Epidemic: Magic Bullets, Psychiatric Drugs, and the Astonishing Rise of Mental Illness in America*. New York: Crown Publishers.
Whitaker, R., and Cosgrove, L. (2015) *Psychiatry Under the Influence: Institutional Corruption, Social Injury, and Prescriptions for Reform*. New York: Palgrave Macmillan.
Wilkinson, R., and Pickett, K. (2010) *The Spirit Level: Why Equality is Better for Everyone* (rev. ed.). London: Penguin.

Williams, J. B. W., Gibbon, M., First, M. B., Spitzer, R.L., Davies, M., Borus, J., Howes, M. J., Kane, J., Pope Jr., H. G., Rounsaville, B., and Wittchen, H.-U. (1992) 'The Structured Clinical Interview for DSM-III-R (SCID): II. Multisite Test-Retest Reliability', *Archives of General Psychiatry*, 49(8): 630–636.

World Health Organization. (2003) *Investing in Mental Health*. Geneva: World Health Organization.

World Health Organization. (2013) *Mental Health Action Plan 2013–2020*. Geneva: World Health Organization.

2

Marxist Theory and Mental Illness: A Critique of Political Economy

Over the past 35 years, social theory has largely disappeared from scholarship on mental illness. In sociology and related disciplines, critical thinking has been sacrificed in the face of a neoliberal agenda which prioritises "pragmatic" scholarship relevant to current social policy. Consequently, dominant approaches to mental health research do little more than support the contemporary political agenda. Whether big-data epidemiological studies on the levels of "mental illness" within the general population or small in-depth analysis of psychiatric experiences, contemporary research is usually bereft of any problematising of the mental health system, the psy-professions, or the psychiatric discourse on which such professions lay claims to expertise. Shamefully, we have left it largely to those within these professions to raise the most awkward questions on the mental health business including the lack of validity of current mental disorders, the increasing medicalisation of everyday behaviour, the close ties to pharmaceutical companies, and the role of these groups as agents of social control. Too many sociologists are scared of engaging with the critical issues—they fear being labelled as "antipsychiatry" or of denying survivor/user experience, and they worry about being excluded from funding streams if they raise serious issues about the nature and purpose

B.M.Z. Cohen, *Psychiatric Hegemony*,
DOI 10.1057/978-1-137-46051-6_2

of the mental health system in capitalist society. Yet if sociologists of medicine are truly serious about accurately researching issues of health and illness, if we still "care" about our subject area, then there is an urgent need to contextualise our work in a set of historical and contemporary power relations. As Vincente Navarro (1980: 200) has previously made clear,

> The actual way of studying disease in any society is by analyzing its historical presence within the political, economic, and ideological power relations in that specific social formation. And by this, I do not mean the analysis of the natural history of disease but rather the political, economic, and ideological determinants of that disease, determinants resulting from the overall power relations which are primarily based on the social relations of production. These power relations are the ones which determine the nature and definition of disease, medical knowledge, and medical practice.

This book is my contribution to reigniting critical thinking within the sociology of mental health.

This chapter begins by outlining the Marxist theory of "materialism," a critique of the political economy of capitalist society which aims to explain economic and social disparities as a historical process. An understanding of Marxist theory allows us to view capitalism as an economic system of fundamental inequalities which are reproduced not only in activities specifically related to the exchange of labour and commodities but rather in all aspects of social, cultural, and political life. In other words, capitalism frames institutional, group, and personal understandings of the world and responses to it. This includes the structure, practices, and priorities of the mental health system itself—an issue which is discussed with reference to those scholars who have previously applied Marxist theory to medicine and psychiatry including Navarro, Waitzkin, Brown, and Parker. Following these scholars, I spend the remainder of the chapter performing a Marxist assessment of the political economy of the mental health system. This is done through analysing a range of colourful and horrific socio-historical examples—including tranquilizer chairs, masturbation, lobotomies, vibrators, shock treatment, and a lot of drugs—to demonstrate how psychiatry and allied professions have served the needs of capitalism both economically and ideologically.

Historical Materialism

Karl Marx's analysis of capitalism is recognised by scholars on both the right and the left as highly significant in explaining the formation and continuance of the fundamental economic and social inequalities witnessed within advanced industrial societies. His theory of historical materialism states that the source of human progress and historical change is not to be found in "legal relations" or "political forms," but rather "in the material conditions of life" (cited in Howard and King 1985: 4). By this Marx means that the economic relations of human beings determine all other relations in that society. Material survival rather than the development of rationality and spiritual thinking forms the fundamental basis of human endeavour in each historical epoch (Palumbo and Scott 2005: 42). In challenging the individualist, liberal theorising of many of his contemporaries, Marx argued that industrial society had not created a radically new society of rational individuals endowed with free will, but instead introduced a new form of industrial slavery which in many ways replicated the medieval serfdom of feudal society. "Freedom" in industrial society is thus an illusion created by a more complex set of societal relations in which political and legal institutions—designated by Marx as part of the "superstructure" of capitalism—reproduced and reinforced these economic relations as appropriate and just. In explaining this contention, Marx (cited in Howard and King 1985: 5, emphasis added) argues,

> In the social production of their existence, men inevitably enter into definite relations, which are independent of their will, namely relations of production appropriate to a given stage in the development of their material forces of production. The totality of these relations of production constitutes the economic structure of society, the real foundation, on which arises a legal and political superstructure and to which correspond definite forms of social consciousness. *The mode of production of material life conditions the general process of social, political and intellectual life.* It is not the consciousness of men that determines their existence, but their social existence that determines their consciousness.

For Marx, the mode of production in any given epoch consists of the *forces of production* (technologies, raw materials, and so on) and the *relations of production* entailing "forms of social organized labour based on the laws of ownership" (Palumbo and Scott 2005: 44). The relations of production determine the status and social-class position of the population dependent on whether they are the owners—the ruling classes, or "bourgeoisie"—or the workers—the working classes, or "proletariat"—of the means of production (in this case, factories, offices, businesses, and so on). Unique to capitalist society, the means of production are privately owned, with the goal of the ruling classes to accumulate and maximise profit through a competitive and expanding market for commodities (Palumbo and Scott 2005: 45). Capitalist society is therefore marked by a fundamental disparity in the distribution of economic resources between the majority of the population—the working classes—who are only "free" to sell their labour to the bourgeoisie, and the small elite who own and control the economic base. It is a system of exploitation in which the workers generate "surplus value" for the ruling classes from their labour, are alienated from what they produce, and in turn are commodified by this process (Palumbo and Scott 2005: 46). The workers are kept at subsistence wages, while the elite accumulate greater wealth—the rich will get richer, prophesied Marx, while the poor will get poorer. Though this has not precisely been the case as industrial capitalism has progressed, there is still plenty of evidence for the continuance of huge inequalities in income and wealth in western society, as well as increasing of gaps between the rich and the poor since the emergence of neoliberalism 35 years ago (see, e.g., Organisation for Economic Co-operation and Development 2015).

On this basis, Marx conceptualises capitalist society as chaotic, anarchic, and riddled with contradictions. Ultimately, it is a system defined by the permanent struggle between the proletariat and the bourgeoisie over the means of production—a conflict which the workers are destined to win through uprising and revolution, eventually creating a new socialist or communist society defined by common ownership and an equal distribution of resources based on need (Crossley 2005: 291). It is "one of the contradictions of capitalism," Brown (1974: 17) notes, "that as capitalism creates a working class that it then exploits, the development of that class seals the fate of the capitalist system, for the working class will overthrow the bourgeois class." Within capitalist society lies the seed of its own destruction. The conflict between the social classes will come to a conclusion when the working classes reach "class consciousness"—that is, a recognition of their true social and economic existence under capitalism. However, in the meantime, Marx argued that the exploitative conditions of capitalism led to the alienation of workers from their social environment. The natural sociability and communality of the people is displaced by the brutality of lived conditions under capitalism (Palumbo and Scott 2005: 47). Marx theorised that the workers had exchanged "relations between persons into relations between things," a "commodity fetishism" in which objects instead of social relations embody worth and value (Palumbo and Scott 2005: 47). This was one form of "false consciousness" of the working classes, a process of exchanging awareness of the true nature of capitalism for the false values of commodities, a part of ruling class ideology. This ideology of capitalism is perpetuated by the superstructure and institutions of civil society such as the church, the state, the criminal justice system, the education system, the media, and the health system.

The next section draws on the Marxist understandings of historical materialism to explore how these ideas can be applied to the field of medicine and psychiatry. My contention is that the priorities and practices of the western health care system facilitate capitalist goals in two distinct ways: first, through direct and indirect profit accumulation, and second, through the social control of deviant populations and the ideological reproduction of dominant norms and values of the ruling classes.

Marxism, Medicine, and Mental Health

Many years ago when the Channel Tunnel—connecting England and France—was being built (1986–1992), I got the chance to talk to a nurse working on the project on the English side. The project was big, deadlines were tight, and the workers, she told me, were suffering terrible conditions in the tunnel (a total of ten workers died during the construction (Smith 2015)). I wondered how complicated her job was as part of the onsite health personnel for such a large project. Not very. "The men mostly come to me complaining of terrible headaches," she explained, "my job is to give them two aspirin and get them back down the tunnel as quickly as possible."

Speaking of medicine under capitalism, Waitzkin (2000: 37) notes the fundamental contradiction between the perception of health as the ultimate "caring profession" and a society which establishes obstacles to the goal of alleviating "needless suffering and death," for "[t]he social organization of medicine also fosters patterns of oppression that are antithetical to medicine's more humane purposes. These patterns within medicine mirror and reproduce oppressive features of the wider society as well." Marxist scholars of medicine have theorised this replication of the wider class struggle within the health system in a number of ways. First, the priorities of the institution favour those of capitalism and the ruling class. For example, the modern system of health care emerged out of the need for a healthier and more reliable industrial workforce (Waitzkin 2000: 48); concern for the health of the working classes has tended to peak when there are imperialist wars to be fought, while the majority of current medical research prioritises lifestyle and "me too" cosmetic treatments for the global market rather than research on life-saving treatments for cancer and infectious diseases (see, e.g., Rapaport 2015). Second, the exploitative work relations within capitalist societies are replicated within the rigid hierarchy of medicine, with high-waged, upper middle-class consultants holding a great amount of decision-making power at the top, the lower middle-class nursing managers administering consultants' needs in the middle, and—holding no power whatsoever and subject to the whims of health managers—the low-earning working-class orderlies and auxiliary staff at the bottom of the pyramid. Navarro (1976: 446) also notes the tendency of the medical profession to maintain and reinforce these class relations through "both the distribution of skills and knowledge and the control of technology" within the health service. Third, the health system functions as an institution of social control. That is, it reinforces the dominant values and norms of capitalism through its surveillance and labelling practices. In the words of Freidson (1988: 252), medicine acts as a "moral entrepreneur" to the extent that illness is viewed negatively and as something to be "eradicated or contained." Even cancer, he states, is a *social valuation* by the profession, a moral rather than an objective judgement of the body, even if it is one "on which most people happen to agree" (Freidson 1988: 252). Taking a Marxist approach to medicine includes recognising the policing function of the health professions to label and "medicalise" social deviance as illness, as well as reinforce the ideological prerogatives of capitalism as natural and common sense (for instance, through biomedical interventions focused on the individual rather than the wider social environment).

The social control function within psy-professional work practices and knowledge claims is reasonably easy to identify and has been a major focus of critical scholars—Marxist and otherwise—since the 1960s (see, e.g., Conrad 1975; Goffman 1961; Rosenhan 1973; Scheff 1966). The moral judgements that mental health experts make of people's behaviour under the claims of scientific neutrality and objectivity allow them to sanction forms of deviance which run contrary to the prevailing social order. For example, Szasz (cited in Freidson 1988: 249) stated in 1964 that "agoraphobia is illness because one should not be afraid of open spaces. Homosexuality is an illness because heterosexuality is the social norm. Divorce is illness because it signals failure of marriage." Specifically, Marxist contentions of the psy-professions as agents of social control focus on the ways in which these experts contribute to the alienation of people from their own creative abilities. These experts utilise their knowledge claims on human behaviour to depoliticise attempts at social transformation at the group and community level, in turn acknowledging only individual solutions as possible. Consequently, states Parker (2007: 2), this "psychologisation of social life" performed by mental health workers "encourages people to think that the only possible change they could ever make would be in the way they dress and present themselves to others."

Ultimately, however, a Marxist critique of political economy needs to consider the ideological function in the context of the underlying economic prerogatives of capitalism. The social control of populations considered as deviant and labelled as "mentally ill" by the psy-professions serves specific requirements of the market, whether this is through the profiteering from individual treatments, the expansion of professional services, or the reinforcement of work and family regimes in the name of appropriate treatment outcomes. In his critical work on the history of psychiatry, Scull (1993: 10) argues that the emergence of the psychiatric profession can be explained as a result of the changes in the social organisation of deviance brought about by new market relations. He asserts that the rise of industrial society required a more complex response to social deviance; there was especially a need to adequately control such groups—who were no longer tied to the land, but instead "free" to sell their labour to the emerging bourgeois—and separate the non-able bodied (e.g., the sick, disabled, poor, alcoholic, vagrant, and elderly) from the "healthy" population. Thus, the growth of the asylums for "the mad" is understood as an economically efficient means by which groups of deviants could be physically separated from the rest of society and kept under close surveillance by new professional authorities (Scull 1993: 33). In Scull's (1993: 29) words,

> the main driving force behind the rise of a segregative response to madness (and to other forms of deviance) can … be asserted to lie in the effects of a mature capitalist market economy and the associated ever more thoroughgoing commercialization of existence.

Therefore, it is ultimately the goals of capitalism which directs industrial society's response to social deviance and, in this way, brings about the formation of the medical attendants/mad doctors/alienists who would in time become the psychiatric profession.

A Marxist approach to understanding the mental health system necessarily has to analyse professional organisation, discourse, and practice, at both the economic and ideological levels. As Brown (1974: 17–18, emphases original) remarks, a Marxist approach to the psy-professions helps us make sense of "*the manifestation, on a huge, technological basis, of capitalist economic relations*," so we can then "*understand the role of psychology and psychiatry as mediating the economic-class structure and the personal emotional structure.*" Psychiatry's claims to "scientific practice," remarks Scull (1993: 392–393), means it has "great potential value in legitimizing and depoliticizing efforts to regulate social life and to keep the recalcitrant and socially disruptive in line." However, this medicalisation of deviance by the mental health experts should not be treated as fundamentally distinct and separate from the economic base that determines the specific form—as well as the groups—who are regulated under such regimes of power. As Parker (2014: 167) states of psychotherapy, a Marxist analysis allows us to understand the profession within capitalism "as an apparatus that not only participates in the production of value but also … [becomes] more important to the production, circulation and management, in both the State and civil society, of subjectivity." In this manner, the following section will analyse a range of examples from the history of psychiatry, highlighting both their specific techniques for managing subjectivity as agents of social control and the production of economic value from their operations.

Industrialisation and the Mad Doctors

Official historians of psychiatry see Philippe Pinel's unchaining of the mad in Paris in 1793 as a highly symbolic moment when the insane were, for the first time, recognised as human beings in need of therapeutic intervention rather than imprisonment and mistreatment (see, e.g., Lieberman 2015: 35–36). It is the formal beginning of the psychiatric profession, a new group of medical experts whose vocation will be to care for and treat the mentally ill as opposed to punish them. Pinel's *traitement moral* (known in the Anglo-American world as "moral treatment" or "moral therapy") was hailed as a truly humanitarian approach to the management of the mad which reflected the rationalism of the new industrial world. Rather than forwarding an organic aetiology for madness, patient case studies suggested to Pinel that particular life events or trauma was at the root of their disturbed behaviour. It was felt that "moral" means could correct the actions of the insane through a more understanding response involving listening to patient complaints, reasoning with them, and showing kindness (Porter 2002: 104). Pinel's philosophy placed an emphasis on the humane care of the insane with the goal of returning them to "rationality" and good health through respectful, therapeutic discourse. His own commentaries on moral treatment, however, cautioned that "successful treatment depended on the employment of psychological terror and fear to gain the compliance of the insane" (Kirk et al. 2013: 45). This importance placed on threats, compliance, and the reform of character found at the very birth of psychiatric practice is something that we continue to see in the "therapeutic" setting today. Fundamental here is the emergence of new understandings of madness which closely align with the changing forces of production and the management of social deviance. Psychiatry's success is dependent on the profession's usefulness in serving the industrial order, including the demands of the bourgeoisie for a highly regulated and compliant workforce. It is more than coincidence that the profession remains—without any trace of irony—insistent on aligning their earliest developments with the appropriately named system of "moral treatment."

Following Pinel, William Tuke and his fellow Quakers implemented the principles of moral treatment at their York Retreat in England. At this rural residence patients were to be treated humanely and with dignity; a minimum of physical restraint was utilised, instead the custodians encouraged various forms of behavioural adjustment. However, transgressions from acceptable standards of "normal" and proper conduct would not be tolerated. Rather than be idle, patients were expected to take up work and hobbies, adhere to good manners at all times, to dress appropriately, and be considerate in social interactions with staff, other patients, and visitors to the Retreat (Foucault 1988a: 241–278). With a ratio of one staff member to every three patients, Tuke claimed a 70 per cent recovery rate among patients at the establishment (Whitaker 2010b: 24).

Contemporary commentators continue to see moral treatment and the practices at the York Retreat as examples of what good mental health care should be (see, e.g., Borthwick et al. 2001). Its underlying philosophy, however, reflected wider puritanical responses of Victorian society to the socially deviant. A reform of character under industrial capitalism was not only desirable but also necessary; by force of will, the irrational citizen would now be made rational again. As Foucault (1988a: 241–278) has discussed, moral treatment was a shift in the management of those labelled as "mad" in as much as the new disciplinary apparatus enforced a closer surveillance of personal conduct, so as to instil obedience to authority in a new set of societal relations. Kirk et al. (2013: 45) have noted of the Retreat that it was still an institution that confined people against their will and utilised a system of rewards and punishments to enforce "psychological and physical conformity." Making progress in this system of moral treatment, state Kirk et al. (2013: 45),

> required obedience and proper behavior by the patients. Failure to follow the rules dramatically undermined the patient's social status, institutional privileges, and personal wellbeing by the forced transfer to more remote and less respectable and comfortable wards. Total control by the alienists/moral managers over the physical and social environment of the inmates was the mechanism that imposed discipline.

This moral management of social deviance was appropriated and replicated by the medical attendants/mad doctors in the larger asylum system over the course of the nineteenth century. Mass incarceration in such facilities effectively facilitated, "sweeping from the streets the poor, the indigent, the mad and the homeless, [and] unsightly beggars" (Breggin 1993: 145), yet at the same time offered a philosophy of care and treatment which emphasised humanitarianism and the potential for recovery. Effectively, the mad doctors succeeded in gaining jurisdiction over the mentally ill through a convincing medical rhetoric on mental disease, even though, as Abbott (cited in Kirk et al. 2013: 9) notes, "[o]f its treatments, only incarceration had any effect, and that made the psychiatrists little different from the jailers they had replaced, despite their reference to the medical model of science, treatment and cure."

The custodians of the emerging asylum system offered a more sophisticated form of social control consistent with the complexities of the industrial order. It is interesting in this respect that the early proponents of moral treatment were religious orders from whom the mad doctors/alienists appropriated their methods—a move from religion to psychiatry as the moral authority for the scientific age. As Abbott (1988: 298) further comments, the early success of the profession is based on its promise to adjust individuals to the new social order. "From its first interest in prevention and indeed from the moral therapy era," he writes (Abbott 1988: 298, emphasis added),

> psychiatry had been fascinated by the relation of the individual to society. The psychiatric concept of prevention attributed nervous and mental disease to failure of adjustment between individual and society, and assumed successful adjustment would prevent disease. *Adjustment underlay every application of psychiatry to social control; young people must be adjusted to the orderly world, soldiers must be adjusted to trench warfare, workers must be adjusted to factories.*

Foucault (1988b: 180) reiterates Abbott's point when he states that "[f] rom the outset, psychiatry has had as its project to be a function of social order." The mad doctors' control of jurisdiction over those labelled as "insane" was only possible through constructing a medical narrative which reflected and responded to the social and economic concerns of the ruling elites. This is further stressed by Foucault (1988b: 180–181, emphasis original) when he puts himself in the shoes of the alienist/psychiatric profession as they emerge in the nineteenth century;

> everywhere society is meeting a mass of problems, in the street, at work, in the family, etc. – and we psychiatrists are *the* functionaries of social order. It is up to us to make good these disorders. We have a function in public hygiene. That is the true vocation of psychiatry. And that is its true context, its destiny.

A useful example of psychiatry's expanding moral role with industrial society can be seen in Fig. 2.1 which shows an original record of incarceration for the Trans-Allegheny Lunatic Asylum (in the city of Weston, West Virginia), from when it opened in 1864 until 1889. Reasons for admission include "bad whiskey," "desertion by husband," "immoral life," "laziness," "novel reading," "politics," and "uterine derangement".

In the name of "public hygiene," behaviour considered as deviant or threatening to the industrial elites was pathologised by the mad doctors. This included what Szasz (2000: 35) refers to as one of "the most commonly diagnosed and most enthusiastically treated mental disease[s] in the history of medicine," namely masturbatory insanity. As the label suggests, the profession theorised that masturbation was not only an unhygienic and deviant behaviour but one which led to insanity and even suicide (Szasz 2000: 36). Still being offered for the "sufferer" as late as the 1930s, treatment options included "restraining devices and mechanical appliances, circumcision, cautery of the genitals, clitoridectomy, and castration" (Szasz 2000: 36). Widely recognised as the founder of British psychiatry, Henry Maudsley was particularly vocal in his disdain for those engaging in such behaviour; "[t]he sooner [the masturbator] sinks to his degraded rest," opined Maudsley (cited in Szasz 2000: 36), "the better for the world which is well rid of him." This example allows us to identify specific economic and ideological concerns of the ruling classes embedded

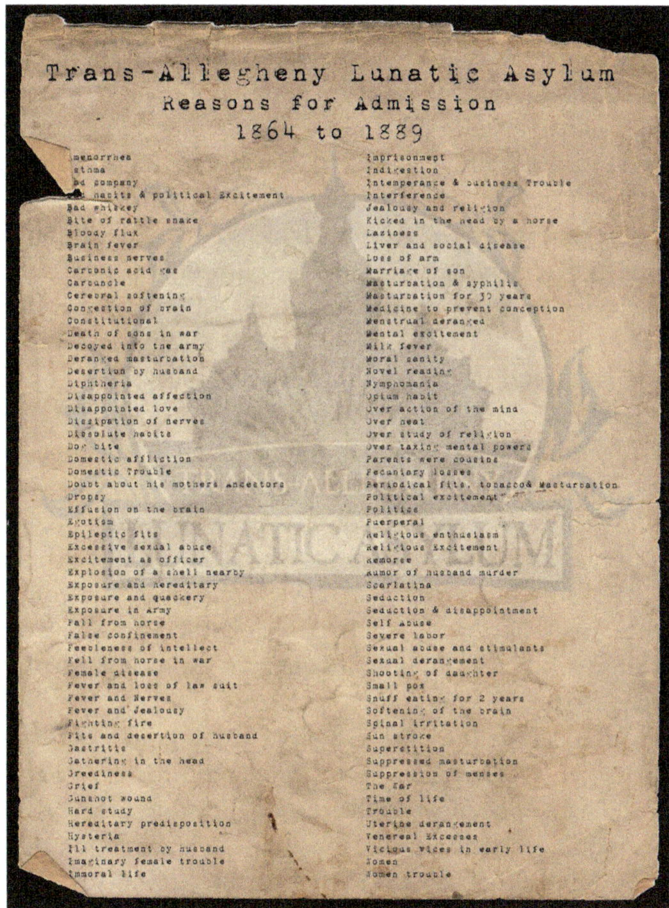

Trans-Allegheny Lunatic Asylum
Reasons for Admission
1864 to 1889

menorrhea
sthma
d company
habits & political Excitement
Bad whiskey
Bite of rattle snake
Bloody flux
Brain fever
Business nerves
Carbonic acid gas
Carbuncle
Cerebral softening
Congestion of brain
Constitutional
Death of sons in war
Decoyed into the army
Deranged masturbation
Desertion by husband
Diphtheria
Disappointed affection
Disappointed love
Dissipation of nerves
Dissolute habits
Dog bite
Domestic affliction
Domestic Trouble
Doubt about his mothers ancestors
Dropsy
Effusion on the brain
Egotism
Epileptic fits
Excessive sexual abuse
Excitement as officer
Explosion of a shell nearby
Exposure and hereditary
Exposure and quackery
Exposure in army
Fall from horse
False confinement
Feebleness of intellect
Fell from horse in war
Female disease
Fever and loss of law suit
Fever and Nerves
Fever and Jealousy
Fighting fire
Fits and desertion of husband
Gastritis
Gathering in the head
Greediness
Grief
Gunshot wound
Hard study
Hereditary predisposition
Hysteria
Ill treatment by husband
Imaginary female trouble
Immoral life
Imprisonment
Indigestion
Intemperance & business Trouble
Interference
Jealousy and religion
Kicked in the head by a horse
Laziness
Liver and social disease
Loss of arm
Marriage of son
Masturbation & syphilis
Masturbation for 30 years
Medicine to prevent conception
Menstrual deranged
Mental excitement
Milk fever
Moral sanity
Novel reading
Nymphomania
Opium habit
Over action of the mind
Over heat
Over study of religion
Over taxing mental powers
Parents were cousins
Pecuniary losses
Periodical fits, tobacco& Masturbation
Political excitement
Politics
Puerperal
Religious enthusiasm
Religious Excitement
Remorse
Rumor of husband murder
Scarlatina
Seduction
Seduction & disappointment
Self abuse
Severe labor
Sexual abuse and stimulants
Sexual derangement
Shooting of daughter
Small pox
Snuff eating for 2 years
Softening of the brain
Spinal irritation
Sun stroke
Superstition
Suppressed masturbation
Suppression of menses
The War
Time of life
Trouble
Uterine derangement
Venereal Excesses
Vicious vices in early life
Women
Women trouble

Fig. 2.1 Reasons for Admission to the Trans-Allegheny Lunatic Asylum, 1864–1889

in the construction of the mental illness. As Szasz (2000: 35) has noted, masturbation was useful to psychiatric expansionism insofar as the "disorder" could be potentially applied to the entire population. Children and adults, males and females could all be caught in the masturbatory insanity net; the classification was a clear case of the mad doctors medicalising deviant behaviour. It was also a good example of the expansion of psychiatric jurisdiction through the medicalisation of sex and sexualities.

Further, it is possible to discern here more specific needs to reinforce the family unit as well as productivity within the labour force. As White (2009: 20–21) has outlined, the claimed physical manifestations of masturbatory insanity (including baldness, stammering, blindness, and skin disease) were used as "a means of social control over the activities of men" (White 2009: 21). Sexual activity was to be confined to reproduction; masturbation was associated with an idleness that would not be tolerated in industrial society. Additionally, the burgeoning of ideas on eugenics—avidly taken up by psychiatry (Chap. 7)—suggested that the alleged greater susceptibility of the working classes to insanity was the result of an evolutionary trend which would continue unless abated by compulsory sterilisation of the "mad." Castration for masturbatory insanity was therefore theorised as "hygienic" in halting the reproduction of "inferior stock." For example, the well-known Pennsylvanian gynaecologist, William Goodell, was of the opinion in 1882 that "sound policy" in the future would be "to stamp out insanity by castrating all the insane men and spaying all the insane women," a view shared by the editor of the *Texas Medical Journal* who also believed that the "treatment" would have the additional benefit of stopping insane men from masturbating (cited in Whitaker 2010b: 57–58).

Women who deviated from their primary roles as wives, mothers, and homemakers were a particular target for the masturbatory insanity label. In the second half of the nineteenth century, the profession began specialising in female "mental illnesses" such as hysteria and nymphomania. The prerogatives of industrial capitalism dictated that a woman's place was in the home, and psychiatry reinforced these patriarchal norms through the social control of women who deviated from the prescribed gender role (Chap. 5). Isaac Baker Brown of the Obstetrical Society of London, for example, was a firm believer that female madness was primary caused by masturbation, suggesting that symptoms could be detected in those women who desired work and were indifferent to their domestic obligations (Showalter 1980: 176–177). From 1859, he performed clitoridectomies on women and girls (as young as ten years old) for a variety of deviations including a 20-year old who disobeyed her mother and was a serious reader, a woman who was "forward and open" with men and had never had an offer of marriage, and a unmarried dressmaker with digestive problems (Showalter 1980: 177). Brown's surgical mutilations were particularly recommended for uncooperative wives, with Showalter (1980: 177) noting that he "urged clitoridectomy for women seeking divorce and believed that the operation would make them more contented, and certainly more manageable, wives." It is recorded that this specific surgical intervention did not vanish from asylums until the 1950s (Whitaker 2010b: 79).

In another ironic twist in the history of mental illness, at the same time as psychiatry was utilising radical interventions to stop disobedient women from masturbating and gaining sexual pleasure outside of the confines of heterosexual marriage, there were colleagues in private practice who—in the name of psychiatric treatment and advances in medicine—were masturbating their "frigid" and matrimonially unsatisfied "hysterical" patients to orgasm. As Maines (1999) has outlined, the "treatment" of middle-class women labelled as "hysterical" was highly profitable for the profession and one which was assisted at the end of the nineteenth century by the introduction of a new "medical aid" and future sex toy, the vibrator. Though seemingly contradictory, both practices can be understood as part of the various attempts by psychiatry to pathologise and control the female body through preserving the status quo of family, marriage, and the industrial division of labour (Chap. 6).

Biological Theory and Physical Treatments

As with prisons and workhouses, institutions for those labelled as "mentally ill" expanded considerably over the course of the nineteenth century in the United Kingdom and the United States. Private clinics and practices for middle-class clients grew and diversified as the century progressed, while large publically funded asylums were built and filled with the working classes. In 1850, there were only 7140 people (4.03 per 10,000 of population) in public asylums in the UK, yet by 1954 there were 148,000 (33.45 per 10,000 of population) (Scull 1984: 67). Similar increases were witnessed in the United States, with over 550,000 people incarcerated in psychiatric institutions by 1955 (Lieberman 2015: 154). In the mid-nineteenth century, the poor for the first time outnumbered the rich as psychiatric patients (Burstow 2015: 38). Private practice individualised social problems of industrial society as various forms of "neuroses"—especially useful in reinforcing the restricted roles of middle-class women. In contrast, the asylum system utilised various physical "treatments" on groups considered as deviant, problematic, or "unfit" to be let loose in wider society. As Scull (1989: 243) notes, with the introduction of state provision, lower-class families were particularly prone to committing troublesome and decrepit family members to the asylum due to the lack of "resources for coping with the dependant and economically unproductive." Thus, as industrial society progressed in the nineteenth century, so business and prestige for the emerging mental health profession flourished.

However, then as now, there remained problems for the alienists/psychiatrists in constructing a valid knowledge base with which to legitimate and justify such expansion to other branches of medicine (as well as the general public). Another major paradox from the history of psychiatry, highlighted by Scull (1989: 239–249), is that as the numbers of the "insane"—measured by the rates of psychiatric incarceration—increased throughout the nineteenth and into the twentieth century, "curability" rates—measured by the numbers discharged from such facilitates—declined. Between the 1870s and the 1920s, the "recovery" rate in England dropped from 40 to 31 per cent (Shorter 1997: 191). Many inmates were incarcerated in such facilities for the entirety of their lives, with Scull (1989) acknowledging that, by the 1950s, the average stay in a US state psychiatric hospital was over 20 years. During the hundred years of growth in the business of private and public psychiatry between 1850 and 1950, colleagues in other branches of medicine had made considerable advances in their knowledge base. In comparison, the mental health experts had made no noticeable progress. This was in spite of psychiatry developing a wide range of biomedical, physically based treatments for mental disorder, some of which will now be discussed.

From the end of the eighteenth century, western medicine made specific advances in their activities due to the appropriation of the language and techniques of scientific enquiry. Impressionistic theories of disease that had been based on the idea of "humoral balance" (Scull 2015: 28) were no longer acceptable in a society built on rationalism and science.

This was encapsulated in Rudolf Virchow's development of the medical "gold standard" for discovering and accurately classifying disease. As Burstow (2015: 36, emphasis original) outlines,

> According to this new understanding, pain or discomfort per se no longer sufficed for something to qualify as a disease. Real *lesion*, real *cellular pathology* observable directly or by tests was to be the standard. While disease might be hypothesized and temporarily entertained in the absence of pathology, to be clear, it was discoveries of pathology alone which confirmed them.

Attempts by the alienist/psychiatric professionals to similarly legitimise their ideas and practices following Virchow's gold standard of medicine are encapsulated in the observational and classificatory work of the German psychiatrist Emil Kraepelin—considered as the "father of modern psychiatry" (Cohen 2014a: 440)—in the latter half of the nineteenth century. Kraepelin's close observations and recording of life histories of over a thousand incarcerated asylum patients led him to theorise that mental disease was caused by discrete, physical entities that incapacitated the normal working of the brain. He developed successive editions of the *Textbook of Psychiatry* (Lehrbuch der Psychiatrie) which outlined his findings and delineated different varieties of mental disorder, including his original descriptions of praecox (later relabelled as schizophrenia) and manic-depression (Cohen 2014a: 440–441). Thus, Kraepelin's work was a successful attempt to promote the idea of a "scientific psychiatry"—that is, a branch of medicine which followed the scientific method and biological theory of their colleagues in other sub-disciplines. As a result of his work, mental disease was firmly established as a disease of the brain, and various treatments aimed at this human organ were progressed under a scientific ethos of hypothesis testing, experimentation, and evaluation. Only one omission from Virchow's gold standard continued to haunt the psychiatric profession, and that was the absence of the discovery of any definite physical pathology. Theories could be entertained, according to Virchow, but not confirmed without real evidence of mental disease. As with those who followed him, Burstow (2015: 43) notes that Kraepelin's ideas on mental pathology hung on assumptions—rather than definite proof—of linkage "between symptoms, etiology, and prognosis." This did not, however, stop psychiatry experimenting on the bodies of those incarcerated in the hope of, retrospectively, proving aetiology.

The physician Benjamin Rush (a signatory to the US Declaration of Independence) was an early believer in the physical aetiology of mental illness. In the 1890s, the man who would become known as "the father of American psychiatry" (his face still appears on the APA emblem) announced his latest cure for madness, the "tranquilizer chair." Whitaker (2010b: 16) explains the workings of this invention,

> Once strapped into the chair, lunatics could not move at all—their arms were bound, their wrists immobilized, their feet clamped together—and their sight was blocked by a wooden contraption confining the head. A bucket was placed beneath the seat for defecation, as patients would be restrained for long periods at a time.

Rush was a man of science, he believed that insanity was caused by the irregular flow of blood vessels in the brain. Thus, he argued that the tranquilizer chair calmed and steadied the blood supply of the insane. The device "binds and confines every part of the body," stated Rush (cited in Whitaker 2010b: 16),

> By keeping the trunk erect, it lessens the impetus of blood toward the brain ... [the tranquilizer chair's] effects have been truly delightful to me. It acts as a sedative to the tongue and temper as well as to the blood vessels.

Along with the bloodletting, cold baths and spinning devices that were then popular in "calming" and "curing" the mad (see Whitaker 2010b: 1–38), Rush's new invention was popular back in the asylums of Europe where the attendants were particularly impressed at how the tranquilizer chair could make the most stubborn of inmates "gentle and submissive" following only one or two days of chair therapy (Whitaker 2010b: 16). These early examples of torture disguised as "treatment" by psychiatry developed further in the early part of the twentieth century as they appropriated physically invasive techniques from other branches of medicine.

As the "curability" rates continued to drop and scientific psychiatry faced mounting challenges from Freud's "dynamic psychiatry"—which appeared to offer more potential for positive mental health outcomes (see Shorter 1997: 145–189)—the desire of the public mental health system for credibility intensified in the first few decades of the twentieth century. At this time, public psychiatry adopted the veneer of general medicine by strategic name changing ("asylums" became "hospitals," "alienists" became "psychiatrists", and so on) as well as appropriating physical apparatus (e.g., ambulances and morgues) and interventions (such as drugs and surgery) from other parts of medicine. As Whitaker (2010b: 73–74) has noted, the new psychiatric treatments were different from previous alienist interventions in that they actually "worked"—through permanently damaging the brain. Indeed, Walter Freeman who popularized the transorbital lobotomy in the United States advocated for the procedure as a part of what he called "brain-damaging therapeutics" (Burstow 2015: 52).

Before thorazine appeared on the market in the 1950s (see discussion below), biomedical psychiatry experimented on the socially deviant with a variety of dangerous drug "treatments." These included various poisons such as camphor and metrazol, as well as insulin administered at very high dosages to invoke seizures and comas in the patient (Whitaker 2010b: 91–96). Purposely taking the patient "to the doors of death" (as one physician put it (Whitaker 2010b: 91)), such treatments were considered a success and carried out widely in the psychiatric institutions of the 1930s and 1940s. The hospital staff observed that the inmates became quieter and more obedient following such "treatment," while the patients themselves lived in palpable terror of further interventions of this nature (Whitaker 2010b: 91). The "treatments" remained dangerous, causing not only brain damage for many but also occasionally death. Meanwhile, some psychiatrists remained concerned that these interventions were less than permanent and did not signify a long-term cure for chronic mental illness.

Two forms of "physical therapy" on the brain that tended to produce more permanent effects (we might say damage) were ECT (more commonly known as "electroshock treatment") and lobotomy. Along with drug treatments, both of these interventions in modified forms are still in use today. Crucial here in understanding the perceived "effectiveness" of these treatments—despite a lack of any evidence for the biological aetiology of mental disease—is to highlight the ways in which they successfully adjusted the behaviour of the socially deviant in a way which allowed for discharge back to the family and even a return to work. The treatments are not an advance in psychiatric medicine, but nevertheless useful in modifying inappropriate behaviour in a more permanent manner, in turn aiding capitalist prerogatives for productivity in the family and the labour force. Both "treatments" would eventually take a back seat to "antipsychotic" drugs, which some scholars argue perform essentially the same task as ECT and psychosurgery in damaging the brain, yet do so in a cheaper and seemingly more effective manner (see, e.g., Breggin 1991; Breggin and Cohen 1999; Moncrieff 2009; Whitaker 2010a).

To understand these physical interventions as forms of social control of deviant groups, it is useful to consider those who were first forced to have the treatments, and the groups who have been subsequently prioritised for them. ECT was first performed in 1938 on an Italian homeless man rounded up by the police in Rome. The inspiration for placing electrodes on the forehead of psychiatric inmates and giving them electric shocks was Italian psychiatrist Ugo Cerletti's visit to a local slaughterhouse where he observed pigs being stunned with electric jolts, making them more manageable for butchers to kill. After being shocked with 110 volts through the brain, Cerletti's first human guinea pig experienced a seizure and subsequently pleaded with the psychiatrist not to inflict the "treatment" on him again (by this point the vagrant was under the—not too surprising—impression that the psychiatrist was going to kill him); Cerletti announced ECT a triumph (Whitaker 2010b: 96–98). Then as now, the procedure produces a convulsion or grand mal seizure (van Daalen-Smith et al. 2014: 206) which appears to "calm" the patient and inhibit the behaviour conceptualised by mental health workers as various forms of "psychoses" or "autism." The psychiatric profession remains baffled as to how ECT works on the body, yet a recent review of the available evidence stated that the only known effects are permanent brain dysfunction and a higher risk of death (Read and Bentall 2010).

As with the drug treatments that preceded it, ECT has been a none-too-subtle method of psychiatric torture which demands conformity from psychiatric inmates, either by threat or as a result of the intervention itself;

as Burstow (2015: 55) reminds us, the Nazi doctors were early adopters of ECT for use on concentration camp inmates. From the earliest experimentations with ECT, it appears that psychiatry was quite aware that electroshock resulted in brain trauma, generally feeling that this was no bad thing. ECT-inflicted patients were observed as experiencing amnesia, being disorientated, lethargic, and apathetic; some noted that their whole intellect was lowered by the "treatment" (Whitaker 2010b: 98). This was all seen as helpful for the patient, for as one physician (cited in Whitaker 2010b: 99) noted, "the greater the damage [to the brain], the more likely the remission of psychotic symptoms."

It was the perceived intellect of the inmate population that particularly marked them out for ECT. Noted pioneer, Dr Abraham Myerson (cited in Burstow 2015: 55), bluntly stated of candidates for ECT that

> [t]hese people have ... more intelligence than they can handle, and the reduction of intelligence is an important factor in the curative process. I say this without cynicism. The fact is that some of the very best cures that one gets are in those individuals whom one reduces almost to amentia [simple-mindedness].

ECT has experienced a recent resurgence, with psychiatrists now keen to target deviant young people labelled as "depressed" or "autistic" for shock treatment if they "fail to respond" to drug interventions (Breggin and Breggin 1998: 195; see also Tomazin 2015; van Daalen-Smith et al. 2014). Leonard Roy Frank (cited in Mills 2014: 93), a survivor of ECT, rhetorically asks, "[w]hy is it that 10 volts of electricity applied to a political prisoner's private parts [genitalia] is seen as torture while 10 or 15 times that amount applied to the brain is called 'treatment'?" Because, I would argue, the threat of ECT is effective in policing those who fail to perform their family, school, work, or consumer roles in western society. Yet, even for some of those in the profession, the treatment remained imprecise as a biomedical intervention and it soon appeared that ECT would be superseded by Egas Moniz's Nobel Prize-winning "miracle cure" of the lobotomy (Whitaker 2010b: 107–108).

Inspired by observations of World War I veterans who had suffered prefrontal brain damage, neurosurgeons suggested that operating on the brains of those labelled as mentally ill could dull the emotions and reduce the intellectual capacity in a more permanent and specific way than ECT had been able to. Egas Moniz theorised that pathological thoughts were "fixed" in the "celluloconnective systems" in the prefrontal lobes of the brain, thus the "cure" for mental disorder was to "destroy" these connections through psychosurgical interventions (Whitaker 2010b: 107–108). Like the majority of subsequent lobotomies, Moniz's first procedure was carried out on a woman (in this case, a former prostitute). As Whitaker (2010b: 113) describes the operation, Moniz "drilled holes into her skull, used a syringe to squirt absolute alcohol onto the exposed white fibers, which killed tissue through dehydration, and then sewed her back up." The woman was subsequently returned to the asylum, where the psychiatrists reported that she remained in a calm state. Following this "successful" operation, further prefrontal operations on the incarcerated population were performed, and by 1936, Moniz was advertising his drilling procedure as demonstrating marked improvements in all of the operated patients (including the observation that post-operative manic-depressives had become "less emotional") (Whitaker 2010b: 114).

During the 1940s and 1950s, Moniz's psychosurgery was made popular in America through the refinements made by Walter Freeman and his neurosurgeon assistant James Watts. Their first patient was again female—a 63-year-old woman who Freeman felt dominated her husband and who he described as a "master of bitching" (cited in Whitaker 2010b: 115). Freeman and Watts were pleased with the results of the operation, writing in the *Southern Medical Journal* that the woman was now able to carry out household chores and appeared to her husband, "more normal than she had ever been" (cited in Whitaker 2010b: 116). By the end of 1936, the physicians had operated on a further 16 women and 3 men (Whitaker 2010b: 116). Post-operative evaluations of patient behaviour were almost exclusively carried out by staff at the psychiatric facilities where the procedures had been performed, focusing on the social norms of "appearance, work, and activity levels" (Getz 2009: 145). Not surprisingly, the results were considered overwhelming positive. Freeman (cited in Getz 2009: 145) himself was especially proud that, as with ECT, intellect and creative functioning was permanently curtailed by the surgical procedure, declaring that "[n]one of our patients has written a book, designed a house, composed a piece of music or invented a salable gadget." The particular targets for lobotomy were the black community as well as uncooperative women. This issue is highlighted in Freeman's own recollections (cited in Burstow 2015: 53–54) of lobotomising a black woman who had been confined in a padded cell at the psychiatric hospital for some years: "when it came time to transfer her … for operation," he recalls,

> five attendants had to restrain her while the nurse gave her the hypodermic [injection]. The operation was successful in that there were no further outbreaks … From that day after … (and we demonstrated this repeatedly to the ward personnel), we could grab [the patient] by the throat, twist her arm, tickle her in the ribs and slap her behind without eliciting anything more than a wide grin and hoarse chuckle.

As with all of psychiatry's physical interventions, the lobotomy "worked" for capitalism in as far as they pacified troublesome groups for good. The left-wing filmmaker and actor Frances Farmer was but one of many political victims of Freeman's psychosurgery. As Ussher (2011: 71; see also Getz 2009: 146) has recounted, Farmer was originally committed to Washington State Hospital by her mother in 1944 for "drinking, smoking, swearing and having sex with men," she was eventually lobotomised and returned home in 1950. The same fate was visited on John F. Kennedy's older sister, Rosemary Kennedy, by her father in 1941, following his concerns for her aggressive behaviour and the fear that she might become pregnant (Getz: 2009: 146; see also Burstow 2015: 54).

Whitaker (2010b: 123) notes that the majority of lobotomised patients were able to leave the hospital, leading to the phrase "lobotomy gets 'em home" becoming popular in the media as news of the "miracle cure" spread. The surgery was increasingly argued to be useful for not only psychotic conditions such as schizophrenia and manic-depression but an ever-widening variety of mental disorders (including anxiety and depression) as well as for dealing with "criminals, psychopaths, and sexual perverts" (Valenstein 1980: 96). The operation was even recommended to American housewives who were finding the tedium of homemaking and childrearing too boring to cope with. As late as 1980, Valenstein (1980:

90) was suggesting that such women remained appropriate cases for psychosurgery. He states of one typical case for the procedure:

> Household chores such as washing-up or polishing a table were completely impossible for her, as they took so long and caused her such distress. Her husband and mother were, therefore, forced into running her home and, on medical advice, her two children were at boarding school.

ECT, antidepressants, and psychotherapy all had a limited effect on this woman's behaviour—each time she "relapsed" after a few weeks—and Valenstein (1980: 90–91) suggested that in such "hard to reach" cases, psychosurgery would still make sense as a part of modern psychiatric treatment. Here we see the continuation of physical therapies as forms of social control; the appropriate gender role for women as mothers and wives being reinforced through the "scientific" psychiatric discourse and "treatment" technologies of the mental health system (Chap. 6).

Freeman eventually became frustrated with the amount of time the Moniz-designed brain-drilling operations took and his reliance on an assistant to anesthetise the patient. Instead he devised a simpler, cheaper and less time-consuming operation which he boasted could be done in 20 minutes (Whitaker 2010b: 133). The procedure required no anaesthetic—instead he used three successive shocks of ECT to pacify the patient—and could be administered by any psychiatrist after only a few hours of training. Freeman's infamous "transorbital lobotomy" innovation has been described by Whitaker (2010b: 133) as follows:

> Freeman attacked the frontal lobes through the eye sockets. He would use an ice pick to poke a hole in the bony orbit above each eye and then insert it seven centimeters deep into the brain. At that point, he would move behind the patient's head and pull up on the ice pick to destroy the frontal-lobe nerve fibers.

Freeman (cited in Whitaker 2010b: 133) even felt it unnecessary to sterilise the ice pick and thereby "waste time with that 'germ crap.'"

Consequently, Burstow (2015: 53) notes that Freeman's innovation further increased medical interest in the procedure, due to its ability to maximise "doctor's profits, [reduce] hospital expenses, and dramatically [increase] the number 'served.'" Thanks to the claims of high "curability" attributed to the transorbital lobotomy by the media and medical journals at the time, over 20,000 social deviants in America alone were lobotomised in the 1950s (Whitaker 2010b: 132). Research articles followed the lobotomists' claims in suggesting that the procedure was a painless, minor, low-risk operation which brought about significant improvement in the patient's behaviour. Over time, however, it became clear that what this implied was that the lobotomy made the inmate more manageable for hospital staff. As Burstow (2015: 52) comments on the subjective judgements made of the lobotomised victim, "behaviour presenting less problems for staff [qualified] as 'improvement.' Indeed, people who could once write poetry and now could do little but giggle were being declared better." Whitaker (2010b: 131) agrees, stating that "any change in behavior [of the lobotomised inmate] that resulted in the patients' becoming more manageable (or less of a bother), could be judged as an improvement." It is unsurprising then that, as Getz (2009: 145) remarks, under such conditions the procedure was increasingly used as a form of punishment by psychiatric staff for unruly behaviour or for those who had not been appropriately pacified by doses of ECT. In fact, Freeman was personally convinced that the more the patient resisted his ice-pick therapy, the more necessary it was that they should receive it (Whitaker 2010b: 133).

Similar to the current expansion of drug treatments for ever-younger groups of deviant, Freeman's evangelical zeal for the lobotomy led him to operate on 11 young people in the 1950s, including one just four years old (Whitaker 2010b: 135). Explaining his rational for lobotomising children, he admitted it was simply an easier and more efficient method of behaviour modification. "It is easier," Freeman (cited in Whitaker 2010b: 136) argued, "to smash the world of fantasy, to cut down upon the emotional interest that the child pays to his inner experiences, than it is to redirect his behavior into socially acceptable channels." It was by this point a typical statement of psychiatric arrogance that subsequently left 2 of the 11 lobotomised young people dead (Whitaker 2010b: 136). Eventually, Freeman—a psychiatrist with no formal surgical training or qualifications—had killed too many patients for the medical establishment to accept and was banned from performing any further lobotomies in the late 1960s. It is estimated that over 40,000 psychiatric patients were victims of psychosurgery while it was fashionable in mid-twentieth-century America (Getz 2009: 147). Subsequently, the "curability" claims made by psychiatry were, once again, found to be groundless. An example is offered by Whitaker (2010b: 135) in describing the reasons for the popularity of the procedure at the Stockton State Hospital in California; the lobotomy could turn "resistive, destructive" inmates into "passive" ones (Braslow, cited in Whitaker 2010b: 135). While a useful method of social control, it was no miracle cure for mental illness; it is estimated that 12 per cent of those lobotomised at the hospital died from the procedure (usually through bleeding in the brain), many more were left severely and permanently disabled, and only 23 per cent ever left the hospital (Whitaker 2010b: 135).

As with ECT, the brutality of the lobotomy has not stopped subsequent attempts by the profession to make it popular again. In the political turmoil of the 1970s, psychiatrists suggested that black people should be targeted for psychosurgery (Burstow 2015: 54), while practitioners in the 1980s considered that the intervention might be of benefit for those suffering from anorexia nervosa, ADHD, and autism (Getz 2009: 148). The latest version of psychosurgery is called "neuromodulation" or "deep brain stimulation," and is recommended for those labelled with depression or obsessive-compulsive disorder (Getz 2009: 147).

While the physical treatments outlined above attempted to offer psychiatry a veneer of biomedical progress to legitimate their activities, they can be more accurately understood as instruments of torture and oppression to more efficiently control those considered as problematic and troublesome to capitalist society. Yet Whitaker (2010b: 127–130) also notes that there were important economic motives for the state and the psychiatric profession to continue experimenting on inmates in search of a more efficient way of managing deviant populations. This included the need for a cheaper form of "care" that could be performed outside the hospital system—an intervention which would address the mounting fiscal crisis caused by the continued funding of large psychiatric hospitals. Mythologised as yet another miracle cure for those labelled as "mentally ill," this would eventuate in the popular promotion of drugs (or "psychopharmaceuticals") within the mental health system, which will be discussed in the next section.

The Drugs "Revolution"

Through the maximisation of profits for pharmaceutical corporations, the contemporary popularity for prescribing drugs is perhaps the most obvious and salient example of psychiatry serving the economic base of capitalism. However, this phenomenon can also be understood as the profession performing its ideological role as a part of the superstructure of capitalism, through the continued individualisation of political discontent and management of the population through chemical agents. The past few decades have witnessed a substantial increase in the consumption of psychiatric drugs across western society. For example, in America, the number of children medicated with ADHD-related drugs (chiefly Ritalin) grew from 150,000 at the end of the 1970s to 3.5 million in 2012 (Whitaker and Cosgrove 2015: 91–92). Similarly in the UK, Moncrieff (2009: 3) notes that the prescriptions for antidepressants increased "by 243 % in the ten years up to 2002." The explosion in profits for pharmaceutical companies over this period has been summated by Whitaker (2010a: 320–321):

> In 1985, outpatient sales of antidepressants and antipsychotics in the United States amounted to $503 million. Twenty-three years later, U.S. sales of antidepressants and antipsychotics reached $24.2 billion, nearly a fiftyfold increase. Antipsychotics—a class of drugs previously seen as extremely problematic in kind, useful only in severely ill patients—were the top revenue-producing class of drugs in 2008, ahead even of the cholesterol-lowering agents. Total sales of all psychotropic drugs in 2008 topped $40 billion. Today—and this shows how crowded the drugstore has become—one in every eight Americans takes a psychiatric drug on a regular basis.

As a result of what Burstow (2015: 167) has termed psychiatry's "march to Pharmageddon," there have been concerns from scholars both inside and outside the psy-professions that drug prescribing is getting out of hand. Specific critiques have suggested that mental health experts may be medicalising evermore aspects of our everyday behaviour as mental illnesses (e.g., our "hoarding," drinking, gaming, grieving, gambling, and so on) so as to prescribe us more drugs; that the professional bodies are far too cosy with pharmaceutical companies and have consequently lost sight of their duty of care to their clients; that the potential health harms of long-term drug taking have been neglected in the hype around the latest "miracle pill" appearing on the market (e.g., Whitaker (2010a: 354) notes that those labelled as "mentally ill" are "now dying twenty-five years earlier than their peers"); and that other therapies are being ignored in favour of the quick-fix chemical cure.

This section demythologises the idea of the "chemical cure" for mental illness by concentrating on the changing economic and political goals of capitalism since the mid-twentieth century. This analysis demonstrates that there can never be a "magic bullet" for mental disorder when aetiology has not been established, thus we have to understand drug treatments as a continuation of the biomedical technologies of control I have discussed so far in this chapter. As with other physical interventions, psychopharmaceuticals can also be understood as a further attempt to legitimise the psychiatric profession as a relevant branch of medicine. A critical evaluation of psychotropic interventions then should not focus on their effectiveness in "treating" or "curing" mental disorders, but rather analyse how this metaphorical placebo aids the survival and expansion of the psychiatric profession beyond the asylum walls. This discussion will break with much of the previous scholarship in the area by arguing that the profit-making ventures of biomedical psychiatry—as reflected in the growth of the new psycho-drugs culture—are in fact secondary to capitalism's desire for the closer surveillance, monitoring, and moral management of the general population in neoliberal society, a function that the psy-professions are most suited for.

Official historians of psychiatry view the introduction of the drug chlorpromazine (marketed as thorazine in America) in the 1950s as a turning point of revolutionary proportions in the treatment and care of the mentally ill. Shorter (1997: 246) calls it "the first drug that worked," while in a chapter titled—in the now familiar irony-free fashion of such writers—"Mother's Little Helper: Medicine At Last," Lieberman (2015: 175, emphasis original) argues that chlorpromazine was "the first *psychopharmaceutical* ... a drug providing true therapeutic benefits for a troubled mind." According to such scholars, this is a breakthrough in psychiatric medicine which can be equated "to the introduction of penicillin in general medicine" (Shorter 1997: 255). It is the beginning of "the era of psychopharmacology" (Shorter 1997: 255) which, as biomedical knowledge on the workings of the brain has progressed, we continue to reap the rewards of today. For Lieberman (2015: 178), chlorpromazine is the first drug to specially target and reduce the symptoms of psychoses (such as hallucinations and disorganised thinking). As he explains, the effect of the drug on institutionalised patients was dramatic and lasting: "[n]ow they could return home," he states, "and incredibly, begin to live stable and even purposeful lives. They had a chance to work, to love, and—possibly—to have a family" (Lieberman 2015: 180). Chlorpromazine was also a significant improvement on previous physical therapies (such as ECT and lobotomy) in terms of being "much less dangerous, and easily tolerated by the patients." Just over a year after the drug was approved by the US Food and Drug Administration (FDA) in 1954, Scull (2015: 367) notes that two million people were taking chlorpromazine in America alone. On this basis, the official history of psychiatry suggests that the introduction of chlorpromazine leads to the slow but inevitable end of the asylum era. In the words of Lieberman (2015: 180), "[i]t is no coincidence that the asylum population began to decline from its peak in the United States in the same year Thorazine was released." For Shorter (1997), the triumph of chlorpromazine as the first "antipsychotic" drug represents a breakthrough for the psychiatric profession as important as Pinel unchaining the mad 150 years before—it was proof of the biological causation of mental disease and, just as importantly, a safe treatment modularity with which to control, if not cure, the symptoms of severe mental disorder.

Unfortunately, the above picture of the psychopharmaceutical "revolution" does not stand up to closer scrutiny. The available evidence demonstrates that the drugs were—and continue to be—no more useful than previous physical treatments, either in the sense of proving an underlying biological aetiology for mental illness or in terms of the potential harm posed to patients (see, e.g., Breggin and Cohen 1999; Burstow 2015; Davies 2013; Kirsch 2009; Moncrieff 2009; Whitaker 2010a). As Moncrieff (2009: 1) has outlined,

> there is no real demarcation between previous eras' psychiatric treatments, and the theories that justified them, and our own; that the need to believe in a cure for psychiatric conditions that drove and sustained people's faith in insulin coma therapy, ECT, radical surgery, sex hormone therapy and many other bizarre interventions is the strongest impetus behind the use of modern-day psychiatric drugs.

I argue here that the drugs revolution can be understood as a significant success for welfare capitalism, where institutional costs are transformed into profits for pharmaceutical corporations. At the same time, the decline of the welfare state and rise of neoliberalism in the 1970s eventuate in chemical forms of social control largely replacing the institution and other forms of physical constraint as the more subtle and preferred technology for managing deviance in capitalist society. Initially suspicious of drug therapy, the evidence also suggests that psychiatric professionals in fact remained for some time wedded to the institution as their traditional power base and only belatedly turned to drugs as a technique of legitimating their expansion beyond the asylum walls. Thus, the idea of a "drugs revolution" in the twentieth century can be understood as a myth used to retrospectively legitimate the current, dominant treatment modality within the mental health system and the continuance of the psychiatric profession as the dominant group of experts responsible for defining and "treating" mental illness.

Contrary to psychiatric mythology, the introduction of chlorpromazine to the mental health system happened by accident rather than design, the term "antipsychotic" being later added by pharmaceutical companies to more effectively market the drug to institutional psychiatry and state authorities. Hypothesised as a beneficial anaesthetic for major operations, the drug was originally used by Henri Laborit, a French naval surgeon, for its antihistaminic properties in 1949. The surgeon (cited in Whitaker 2010a: 48) noted that the results of the drug appeared positive in that the patient "felt no pain, no anxiety, and often did not remember his operation." Thus, Laborit felt chlorpromazine offered a potential improvement on barbiturates and morphine, popularly used as pre-operation anaesthetics at the time. At a medical conference in 1951, he further stated that the drug appeared to produce "a veritable medicinal lobotomy," and for this reason might also be of use to psychiatry (Laborit, cited in Whitaker 2010a: 49). The following year, Jean Delay and Pierre Deniker, two prominent French psychiatrists, put the drug to the test on patients they had labelled as "psychotic" at St. Anne's Hospital in Paris (Whitaker 2010a: 49–50). The first patient to be given the drug was a 57-year-old male labourer who had been admitted for "making improvised political speeches in cafes, becoming involved in fights with strangers, and for … walking around the street with a pot of flowers on his head preaching his love of liberty" (Delay, cited in Shorter 1997: 250). After three weeks of chlorpromazine the psychiatrists discharged the patient, observing a new calmness within him. The authorities were impressed with the results of the drug on the asylum population; while still conscious and responsive to the ward staff, the inmates were much more subdued and quiet. As with ECT and pre-frontal lobotomy, the drug produced a more manageable and compliant patient. The psychiatrists wrote triumphantly of the chlorpromazine-drugged patient in 1952 that "he rarely takes the initiative of asking a question" and, further, "does not express his preoccupations, desires, or preference" (Delay and Deniker, cited in Whitaker 2010a: 50).

As a quick and cheap substitute for lobotomy, the drug quickly became popular across asylums in Europe. Hans Lehmann, the physician who is often cited as responsible for the introduction of chlorpromazine to North America, admitted he was intrigued by the claim of the research papers and drugs marketing literature that the drug acted "like a chemical lobotomy" (Shorter 1997: 252). After the implementation of the drug regimen at his Verdun Hospital in Montreal, Lehmann felt chlorpromazine achieved roughly the same results as insulin treatment and ECT but was an improvement on psychosurgery (of which he was an avid supporter) (Moncrieff 2009: 45). The drug, announced Lehmann, was most useful in managing the psychiatric patient in that it produced an "emotional indifference" in the inmate (cited in Breggin 1991: 55). As Breggin (1991: 55) notes, chlorpromazine was not conceptualised by the profession and business promoters as a cure for mental illness or even an alleviator of symptoms, but rather a pacifier of one's character. "We have to remember," stated the psychiatrist E. H. Parsons (cited in Whitaker 2010a: 50–51) in 1955, "that we are not treating diseases with this drug … We are using a neuropharmacologic agent to produce a specific effect."

That effect has been summated by Breggin (1991: 55, emphasis original) as, "[p]atient's don't lose their symptoms, they lose *interest* in them."

Thus, chlorpromazine's success in sedating patients on the ward was hardly a "revolution" in psychiatric practice. Prior to the 1950s, notes Moncrieff (2009: 41), other psychotropics were used extensively by the profession both inside and outside the institution; "[i]npatients were frequently prescribed several different drugs simultaneously," she comments, "and outpatients were also frequently prescribed drugs, mostly barbiturates and stimulants." Unlike today, this drugging of patients was viewed by the profession as something of an embarrassment; psychiatry was all too aware that such chemical interventions were a form of physical control rather than anything that could be considered as "therapeutic" (Moncrieff 2009: 41). At the time, drugs were not seen by the majority of psychiatrists as central to the future of their practice. For this reason, psychiatrists in America remained, for a time, reticent to use chlorpromazine in their institutions for the simple reason that they already had other physical and chemical treatments which acted in roughly the same manner. Further proof that the drug was no "miracle" pill for mental disorder (as the *New York Times* would go on to describe it in the mid-1950s) (Whitaker 2010a: 58) is provided by Scull (2015: 367–368), who observes both that the numbers of patients in asylums were falling in many parts of America prior to the introduction of chlorpromazine in the 1950s and that many European countries witnessed no such reductions in patient numbers until the 1970s—many years after the drug had been introduced there. The impreciseness of the correlation between chlorpromazine and deinstitutionalisation has led Scull and other commentators (see, e.g., Whitaker 2010a: 206–207) to a different conclusion—that fiscal considerations of state legislatures took precedent over any claims to effective treatment or the "curability" of those labelled as mentally disordered. The psychiatric institution was no longer economically viable as a holding place for problematic populations, so the hype created around new "neuroleptic" drugs such as chlorpromazine and the possibility of returning patients to "the community" were used in a way which "allowed governments to save money while simultaneously giving their policy a humanitarian gloss" (Scull 1984: 139). As Lieberman (2015: 179) notes, the American success of chlorpromazine was achieved by the pharmaceutical company Smith, Kline & French, who focused their efforts on state governments through the fiscal arguments of "health economics" and "cost-cutting," rather than promising psychiatry a miraculous cure for mental illness. Together with a successful media campaign (see Whitaker 2010a: 58–61) claiming that chlorpromazine symbolised a "new era of psychiatry," this tactic worked; within a year of launching the drug, Smith, Kline & French's total sales increased by over a third (Moncrieff 2009: 42).

The success of chlorpromazine was therefore not the result of scientific endeavour and the development of ever-more sophisticated psychiatric practice, but instead social and economic forces beyond the profession—namely, institutions as economically unviable forms of social control, the marketing of drugs by pharmaceutical companies, and the eventual need for the expansion of psychiatry as moral managers of the general population. The success was economic not therapeutic; while no disease had been identified or treated with chlorpromazine, pharmaceutical companies recognised that, with deinstitutionalisation, there was now substantial rewards to be made from the business of community-based mental health care. Meanwhile, governments could justify cuts and closures of the asylums and instead fund outpatients and drug treatments as both cheaper and more "effective" public health interventions. In time, the crisis of deinstitutionalisation facilitated the psychiatric profession's increased commitment to the biomedical model and the use of drugs as a primary source of medical legitimation for their continued practice and expansion into other arenas of economic and social life. Drugs aided the professional legitimation of mental health work outside the institution (Moncrieff 2009: 49), and a revised history of the "drugs revolution" was constructed to suggest the natural progression of psychiatry as a branch of scientific medicine.

At first, the post-war expansion of outpatient clinics and community-based mental health teams (often comprising of a variety of social and medical practitioners) appeared to threaten psychiatry's natural position as the ultimate authority on mental illness. Yet the post-institutional turn to biomedicine and drugs became a useful justification for reinforcing the power of the psychiatrists in these new settings. Only the psychiatrist had the power to prescribe and alter the medications of the patient, and with the growing mythology that the drugs were actually effective, it meant that all other treatment options were given secondary importance, subservient to chemical interventions in the community (for an example of this dynamic, see Samson 1995). Thus, Moncrieff (2009: 44) suggests that by the mid-twentieth century psychiatry had become a "sitting duck" for a new treatment with which they could legitimately justify a disengagement from the asylum and an expansion into the world outside. Drugs provided that justification and fitted well with the popular view from other branches of medicine. As Breggin (1991: 55) states of the benefits of drug interventions for psychiatrists,

> the dose could be "titrated"—that is, it could be raised and lowered to obtain the desired effect. As an ostensibly more humane intervention, drug therapy both salved the consciences of psychiatrists and made them feel more like legitimate doctors.

With the development of successive generations of neuroleptics and selective serotonin reuptake inhibitors (SSRIs) such as Prozac, Zoloft, and Paxil, sales have skyrocketed as psychiatric practice has expanded into new arenas of public and private life. The evidence, however, has repeatedly shown that the drugs do not work. For example, an extensive review of both the published and unpublished clinical trials of the "wonder drug" Prozac by the clinical psychologist Irving Kirsch (2009) concluded that it was no more effective than placebo (i.e., dummy pills with no active ingredients) (see also Whitaker 2010a; Whitaker and Cosgrove 2015). Similar findings have been outlined by Moncrieff (2009) in a review of research on various antidepressants and stimulants. "[P]sychiatric drug treatment," she concludes, "is currently administered on the basis of a huge collective myth; the myth that psychiatric drugs act by correcting the biological basis of psychiatric symptoms or diseases" (Moncrieff 2009: 237). It is therefore an impressive success for biomedical psychiatry that, despite the lack of evidence, the idea of "chemical imbalances" in the brains of those diagnosed as "mentally ill"—and psychopharmaceuticals as the "chemical cure"—has gained such traction in both popular and scientific discourse. In the words of Breggin and Cohen (1999: 35), "[n]o psychiatric drug has ever been tailored to a known biochemical derangement," and, "no biochemical imbalances have ever been documented with certainty in association with any psychiatric diagnosis." This is something that psychiatrists have only recently owned up to, with Ronald Pies (cited in Whitaker and Cosgrove 2015: 186), editor-in-chief of the *Psychiatric Times*, admitting in 2011 that "[i]n truth, the 'chemical imbalance' notion was always a kind of urban legend—never a theory seriously propounded by well-informed psychiatrists." An urban legend may be, but nevertheless a biomedical rhetoric that can justify psychiatric intervention and drug treatment as valid medical practice. The psychiatrist Daniel Carlat has freely acknowledged that using the language of "chemical imbalances" at least suggests to patients that psychiatrists know what they are doing. In 2010, Carlat (cited in Whitaker and Cosgrove 2015: 187, emphasis added) declared,

> I say that ["chemical imbalances in the brain"] not because I really believe it, because I know that the evidence isn't really there for us to understand the mechanism. I think I say that because patients want to know something, and they want to know that we as physicians have some basic understanding of what we're doing when we're prescribing medications. *And they certainly don't want to hear that a psychiatrist essentially has no idea how these medications work.*

Whitaker and Cosgrove (2015: 87) have discussed the significant benefits for both big pharma and the psychiatric profession in promoting drug use in the current mental health system. For the drug companies, psychiatry can medically legitimate their products as well as facilitate the expansion of the potential population for their products. In turn, the drug companies legitimate the institution of psychiatry as a "real" (meaning biomedically-based) part of medicine and facilitate the expansion of its areas of research and expertise through various funding and revenue streams. The outcome of this relationship has been fairly predictable—both parties have benefited enormously over time. Pharmaceutical companies continue to maximise their profits while psychiatry's (and, by extension, other psy-professionals') power—as signified by the proliferation of its discourse among the general population—has significantly expanded over the past 35 years.

That said, the expansion of the psy-professions in general and the proliferation of the psychiatric discourse to hegemonic status in neoliberal society cannot be explained by the success of the drug industry alone. This requires further analysis of the ideological role of psy-disciplines, which will be outlined in the next chapter. Suffice here to say that a Marxist analysis of psychiatric power always needs to consider the benefits to capitalism inferred by their changing discourse and practices. And while every part of civil society can serve the economic base, it is the value of such institutions as part of the superstructure which distinguishes them as ultimately relevant and useful to the ruling classes. So whereas we may think of the drugs issue only in terms of the economic prerogatives of capitalism, it is in fact their value as a means of social and ideological control of the population which should be given particular importance here. As Moncrieff (2009: 238) has rightly stated of the dominant biomedical view of psychopharmaceutical interventions as effective treatment for mental illnesses,

> this knowledge has itself become an instrument of psychiatric power. It has facilitated the particular form of social control that is embodied in psychiatric practice, by construing psychiatric constraint as the medical cure of mental disease. It has helped to disperse psychiatric power throughout the population by concealing the moral nature of psychiatric judgements.

From moral treatment to drug treatment, psychiatry's project remains unchanged: their goal is the moral management and behavioural adjustment of populations considered socially deviant, whether unemployed, underproductive, or politically suspect. The intervention of pharmaceutical companies in the process of psychiatric medicalisation needs to be understood as a rather insignificant factor in the general production of the psychiatric discourse. As Horwitz and Wakefield (2007: 182, emphasis original) have commented on biomedical psychiatry's takeover of the DSM in the 1970s, "[t]here is no evidence that pharmaceutical companies had a role in developing *DSM-III* diagnostic criteria." While this statement might be challenged by the DSM-III research of Lane (2007) and others, it is still accurate to conclude that pharmaceutical companies have never been the *originators* of diagnostic categories; this has remained the responsibility of psychiatry (regardless of how far the profession may sometimes appear to be in big pharma's pockets). Thus, while SSRIs and other contemporary psychoactive drugs can be seen as interventions of social control performed by mental health workers, "to restrain individuals from behavior and experience that are not complementary to the requirements of the dominant value system" (Lennard, cited in Conrad 1975: 19), the specific form of behaviour and experience which is considered in need of reform or restraint is still dictated by the psychiatric profession.

Summary

Utilising Marx's theory of historical materialism, it has been argued in this chapter that the modern mental health system is constituted and framed by the social and economic forces of industrial capitalism. Through a socio-historical survey of the practices and philosophies of the mental health experts from moral treatment to psychopharmaceutical interventions, I have demonstrated that the success of the psychiatric professionals is predicated on their knowledge claims aligning with the goals of the ruling classes for subservient and compliant workers. As a part of the superstructure, the mental health system has aided the economic base through the naturalisation of the fundamental inequalities of capitalist society. This ideological role of the psychiatric system works to depoliticise and individualise the realities of existence within the current social order through medicalising deviance and enforcing conformity on suspect groups. Yet as will be discussed in the following chapter, in neoliberal society the ideological role has been extended, resulting in the psychiatric discourse becoming hegemonic. As Burstow (2015: 70) has summated of this expansion,

> Incomparably more people are intruded on, with that number multiplying with every passing day. Surveillance of anyone who has ever seemed in trouble, surveillance of our children, of seniors is now routine. If once upon a time, one would have to appear "deviant" or to exhibit "unusual behaviour" to fall under the auspices of the "system," now normal childhood

qualifies as a disease. Moreover, the intrusion reaches significantly deeper than the shackles of yesteryear, into the inner recesses of the brain. It is as if psychiatry had removed the fetters from the body of the "lunatic" subject only to place more durable ones on everyone's mind.

Bibliography

Abbott, A. (1988) *The System of Professionals: An Essay on the Division of Expert Labor*. Chicago: The University of Chicago Press.

Borthwick, A., Holman, C., Kennard, D., McFetridge, M., Messruther, K., and Wilkes, J. (2001) 'The Relevance of Moral Treatment to Contemporary Mental Health Care', *Journal of Mental Health*, 10(4): 427–439.

Breggin, P. R. (1991) *Toxic Psychiatry: Why Therapy, Empathy, and Love Must Replace the Drugs, Electroshock, and Biochemical Theories of the 'New Psychiatry'*. New York: St. Martin's Press.

Breggin, P. R. (1993) 'Psychiatry's Role in the Holocaust', *International Journal of Risk & Safety in Medicine*, 4(2): 133–148.

Breggin, P. R., and Breggin, G. R. (1998) *The War Against Children of Color: Psychiatry Targets Inner City Youth*. Monroe: Common Courage Press.

Breggin, P. R., and Cohen, D. (1999) *Your Drug May Be Your Problem: How and Why to Stop Taking Psychiatric Drugs*. Cambridge, MA: Perseus Publishing.

Brown, P. (1974) *Towards a Marxist Psychology*. New York: Harper & Row.

Burstow, B. (2015) *Psychiatry and the Business of Madness: An Ethical and Epistemological Accounting*. New York: Palgrave Macmillan.

Cohen, B. M. Z. (2014a) 'Emil Kraepelin', in Scull, A. (Ed.), *Cultural Sociology of Mental Illness: An A-to-Z Guide* (pp. 440–442). Thousand Oaks: Sage.

Conrad, P. (1975) 'The Discovery of Hyperkinesis: Notes on the Medicalization of Deviant Behaviour', *Social Problems*, 23(1): 12–21.

Crossley, N. (2005) *Key Concepts in Critical Social Theory*. London: Sage.

Davies, J. (2013) *Cracked: Why Psychiatry is Doing More Harm than Good*. London: Icon Books.

Foucault, M. (1988a) *Madness and Civilization: A History of Insanity in the Age of Reason*. New York: Vintage Books.

Foucault, M. (1988b) *Politics, Philosophy, Culture: Interviews and Other Writings, 1977–1984*. New York: Routledge.

Freidson, E. (1988) *Profession of Medicine: A Study of the Sociology of Applied Knowledge*. Chicago: University of Chicago Press.

Getz, M. J. (2009) 'The Ice Pick of Oblivion: Moniz, Freeman and the Development of Psychosurgery', *TRAMES: A Journal of the Humanities & Social Sciences*, 13(2): 129–152.

Goffman, E. (1961) *Asylums: Essays on the Social Situation of Mental Patients and Other Inmates*. London: Penguin.

Horwitz, A. V., and Wakefield, J. C. (2007) *The Loss of Sadness: How Psychiatry Transformed Normal Sorrow into Depressive Disorder*. New York: Oxford University Press.

Howard, M. C., and King, J. E. (1985) *The Political Economy of Marx* (2nd ed.). Harlow: Longman.

Kirk, S. A., Gomory, T., and Cohen, D. (2013) *Mad Science: Psychiatric Coercion, Diagnosis, and Drugs*. New Brunswick: Transaction Publishers.

Kirsch, I. (2009) *The Emperor's New Drugs: Exploding the Antidepressant Myth*. New York: Basic Books.

Lane, C. (2007) *Shyness: How Normal Behavior Became a Sickness*. New Haven: Yale University Press.

Lieberman, J. A. (2015) *Shrinks: The Untold Story of Psychiatry*. New York: Little, Brown and Company.

Maines, R. (1999) *The Technology of Orgasm: 'Hysteria,' The Vibrator, and Women's Sexual Satisfaction*. Baltimore, MD: The Johns Hopkins University Press.

Mills, C. (2014) *Decolonizing Global Mental Health: The Psychiatrization of the Majority World*. Hove: Routledge.

Moncrieff, J. (2009) *The Myth of Chemical Cure: A Critique of Psychiatric Drug Treatment* (rev. ed.). Houndmills, Basingstoke: Palgrave Macmillan.

Navarro, V. (1976) 'Social Class, Political Power and the State and Their Implications in Medicine', *Social Science and Medicine*, 10(9): 437–457.

Navarro, V. (1980) 'Work, Ideology and Science: The Case of Medicine', *Social Science and Medicine*, 14(3): 191–205.

Organisation for Economic Co-operation and Development (2015) *In It Together: Why Less Inequality Benefits All*. Paris: OECD Publishing

Palumbo, A., and Scott, A. (2005) 'Classical Social Theory II: Karl Marx and Émile Durkheim', in Harrington, A. (Ed.), *Modern Social Theory: An Introduction* (pp. 40–62). Oxford: Oxford University Press.

Parker, I. (2007) *Revolution in Psychology: Alienation to Emancipation*. London: Pluto Press.

Parker, I. (2014) 'Psychotherapy under Capitalism: The Production, Circulation and Management of Value and Subjectivity', *Psychotherapy and Politics International*, 13(3): 166–175.

Porter, R. (2002) *Madness: A Brief History*. Oxford: Oxford University Press.

Rapaport, L. (2015) 'U.S. Needs to Raise Investment, Shift Medical Research Priorities', *Reuters*, http://www.reuters.com/article/us-health-investment-research-idUSKBN0KN27B20150114 (retrieved on 21 April 2016).

Read, J., and Bentall, R. (2010) 'The Effectiveness of Electroconvulsive Therapy: A Literature Review', *Epidemiologia e Psichiatria Sociale*, 19(4): 333–347.

Rosenhan, D. L. (1973) 'On Being Sane in Insane Places', *Science*, 179(4070): 250–258.

Samson, C. (1995) 'The Fracturing of Medical Dominance in British Psychiatry?', *Sociology of Health and Illness*, 17(2): 245–268.

Scheff, T. J. (1966) *Being Mentally Ill: A Sociological Theory*. Chicago: Aldine.

Scull, A. (1984) *Decarceration: Community Treatment and the Deviant: A Radical View* (2nd ed.). Oxford: Basil Blackwell.

Scull, A. (1989) *Social Order/Mental Disorder: Anglo-American Psychiatry in Historical Perspective*. Berkeley: University of California Press.

Scull, A. (1993) *The Most Solitary of Afflictions: Madness and Society in Britain, 1700–1900*. New Haven: Yale University Press.

Scull, A. (2015) *Madness in Civilization: A Cultural History of Insanity, from the Bible to Freud, from the Madhouse to Modern Medicine*. Princeton: Princeton University Press.

Shorter, E. (1997) *A History of Psychiatry: From the Era of the Asylum to the Age of Prozac*. New York: John Wiley & Sons.

Showalter, E. (1980) 'Victorian Women and Insanity', *Victorian Studies*, 23(2): 157–181.

Smith, O. (2015) 'The Channel Tunnel: 20 Fascinating Facts', *The Telegraph*, http://www.telegraph.co.uk/travel/destinations/europe/france/articles/The-Channel-Tunnel-20-fascinating-facts/ (retrieved on 21 April 2016).

Szasz, T. S. (2000) 'Remembering Masturbatory Insanity', *Ideas on Liberty*, 50: 35–36.

Tomazin, F. (2015) 'Shock Therapy Figures Spiking', *The Age*, http://www.theage.com.au/victoria/shock-therapy-figures-spiking-20150516-gh33pi.html (retrieved on 6 March 2016).

Ussher, J. M. (2011) *The Madness of Women: Myth and Experience*. London: Routledge.

Valenstein, E. S. (1980) 'Who Receives Psychosurgery?', in Valenstein, E. S. (Ed.), *The Psychosurgery Debate: Scientific, Legal, and Ethical Perspectives* (pp. 89–107). San Francisco: W. H. Freeman and Company.

van Daalen-Smith, C., Adam, S., Breggin, P., and LeFrançois, B. A. (2014) 'The Utmost Discretion: How Presumed Prudence Leaves Children Susceptible to Electroshock', *Children & Society*, 28(3): 205–217.

Waitzkin, H. (2000) *The Second Sickness: Contradictions of Capitalist Health Care* (rev. ed.). Lanham: Rowan & Littlefield Publishers.

Whitaker, R. (2010a) *Anatomy of an Epidemic: Magic Bullets, Psychiatric Drugs, and the Astonishing Rise of Mental Illness in America*. New York: Crown Publishers.

Whitaker, R. (2010b) *Mad in America: Bad Science, Bad Medicine, and the Enduring Mistreatment of the Mentally Ill* (rev. ed.) New York: Basic Books.

Whitaker, R., and Cosgrove, L. (2015) *Psychiatry Under the Influence: Institutional Corruption, Social Injury, and Prescriptions for Reform*. New York: Palgrave Macmillan.

White, K. (2009) *An Introduction to the Sociology of Health and Illness* (2nd ed.). London: Sage.

3

Psychiatric Hegemony: Mental Illness in Neoliberal Society

The previous chapter outlined a critique of the political economy of mental illness, focusing on the psy-professionals' support of the economic base from the development of moral treatment and the asylum system in the nineteenth century to the current profiteering from an expanding drugs market. Demonstrating Marx and Engels' (1965: 37) statement that capitalism "must nestle everywhere, settle everywhere, establish connections everywhere," I have shown that the mental health system generates an increasing range of products and services for the market, mirrors the wider division of labour through exploitative work practices, and functions as an institution of social control, policing deviance, and reinforcing exploitative relations within capitalist society as "normal" and common sense.

This chapter, however, gives special attention to the expanding *ideological power* of the psychiatric discourse within neoliberal society. I present here my core rationale for taking a Gramscian approach to understanding this discourse as "hegemonic," that is, an all-encompassing form of knowledge which works to naturalise and reinforce the norms and values of capital through professional claims-making. As was

B.M.Z. Cohen, *Psychiatric Hegemony*,
DOI 10.1057/978-1-137-46051-6_3

highlighted in the last chapter, the mental health system has always had ideological dimensions, yet the recent demands of neoliberal capital have necessitated the expansion of the psychiatric discourse to the point where it has become hegemonic and totalising. Our behaviour, our personalities, our lifestyles, our relationships, and even our shopping trips are now closely observed and judged under this psychiatric hegemony, and we have in turn come to monitor and understand ourselves through this discourse. As Whitaker (2010a: 10, emphasis original) rightly states of these changes,

> Over the past twenty-five years, psychiatry has profoundly reshaped our society. Through its *Diagnostic and Statistical Manual* [the DSM], psychiatry draws a line between what is "normal" and what is not. Our societal understanding of the human mind, which in the past arose from a medley of sources (great works of fiction, scientific investigations, and philosophical and religious writings), is now filtered through the DSM.

The chapter begins by describing the ideological purpose of professional groups such as psychiatry within advanced capitalist societies. In doing so, I draw on the theoretical work of Gramsci, Althusser, and Habermas in conceptualising how such groups within civil society legitimise ruling class ideology through their practices and constructed discourse. This is followed by a discussion of how this ideological critique can be applied to medicine and psychiatry, as well as a review of the processes through which the psychiatric discourse—that is, the totality of ideas (including the language, practices, and treatments) on "mental illness" and "mental health" that psychiatric and allied professions have circulated to the public over the past 200 years—became hegemonic following the "crisis" of psychiatry in the mid-1970s, the construction of the DSM-III in 1980, and the wider development of neoliberal policies. The final part of the chapter discusses some of the contemporary issues which inform the recent increase in "mental illness" self-surveillance and self-labelling behaviour, a situation, I argue, that further demonstrates the existence of psychiatric hegemony.

Hegemony, Ideology, and Professional Power

Given the oppressive economic conditions that workers endure under western capitalism, Marx (1971) prophesied the proletariat revolution as inevitable. This certainly appeared likely with the European and American financial crises of the 1920s and 1930s and, consequently, a rise in political and class consciousness. It was, however, a catastrophic period which western capitalism survived. In this context of failed revolutions, theorising on the superstructure of capital (Chap. 2) became increasingly important to Marxist writers in addressing the "inevitability" question (Heiner 2006: 10–11). Gramsci's (1971) answer to this question was that the ruling classes ultimately survived threats to their authority not through direct "domination" and coercion of the masses but rather by demonstrating "intellectual and moral leadership." It was the latter type of supremacy that constituted what he termed "hegemony," a form of "internal control" which Femia (1981: 24) outlines as "an order in which a common social-moral language is spoken, in which one concept of reality is dominant, informing with its spirit all modes of thought and behaviour." Or as Kellner (2005: 158) has succinctly defined hegemonic power, the "domination by ideas and cultural forms that induce consent to the rule of the leading groups in society." Gramsci argued that the coercive powers of the state (e.g., the army, police, and the judicial system) were comparatively ineffective and fragile in ultimately halting the revolution; instead the capitalist classes had secured a greater chance of survival through hegemonic power—the rule of the bourgeoisie by induced *consent*. As Crossley (2005: 114) has articulated this idea,

> The bourgeoisie must win the hearts and minds of the people, persuading them (without even seeming to do so or to need to do so) that the status quo is natural and inevitable, beneficial for all, and inducing them to identify with it.

Gramsci located the intellectual and moral leadership won by the ruling classes as residing in civil society rather than the state. By "civil society" he meant institutions such as religion, education, the media, and the family, to which Marxist scholars such as Navarro (1986) and Waitzkin (2000) have added the institution of health as a further site of hegemonic power. These civic institutions are much more effective than direct, repressive organs of the state in manipulating the masses due to their perceived detachment from elite control. Hegemonic power is conducted under the guise of objective and neutral institutional practice, though it is in reality nothing of the sort. Instead, intellectuals and professionals are responsible for the legitimation of ruling class ideas within the public sphere, articulating such values as seemingly natural and taken-for-granted knowledge about the world. Thus, Fontana (1993: 140–141) comments that

> the function of intellectuals is not only to create a particular way of life and a particular conception of the world, but also to translate the interests and values of a specific social group into general, "common" values and interests.

What we understand as "normal" and common sense is in fact dominant, capitalist ideas imparted through professional discourse, an issue summated in the famous quote from Marx and Engels that "the ideas of the ruling class are in every epoch the ruling ideas" (cited in Navarro 1980: 196). Althusser (2005: 114) commented that the concept of hegemony offered "a theoretical solution in outline to the problems of the interpenetration of the economic and the political." In other words, it was an effective explanatory device for understanding the survival of the economic base of capitalism despite significant political struggles against the bourgeoisie in every epoch.

Althusser himself extended Gramsci's conceptions of hegemony by developing a specific theory of ideology. Rather than being directly shaped by the economic base, Althusser suggested that institutions of civil society had a degree of autonomy from it that is "neither totally shaped by the economy nor totally autonomous" (Crossley 2005: 150). This can explain why not every decision, behaviour, or practice of an organisation appears to be traceable back to the economic prerogatives of capitalism. This subtlety within Althusser's analysis highlights that hegemonic power is a form of *negotiated* power in which professional groups and institutions can act in semi-autonomous and sometimes oppositional directions to capital. Each institution has its own set of professional priorities, interests, and values to protect from other competing groups, and sometimes this may bring about conflict with the objectives of the ruling elites. In such situations, compromise is necessary so as not to threaten the fundamental economic base and current social order (Freidson 1988; Williams 1977). Discussing the institution of medicine as part of hegemonic relations, Navarro (1989: 198) summarises this issue of professional autonomy as follows:

> Medical knowledge is not produced and reproduced in the abstract but through agents and relations which are bearers of power relations of which class is a determinant one. To say this is not to say that medical and scientific knowledge does not have an autonomy of its own, but that autonomy takes place within a set of power relations which determines not only how medical knowledge is used … but also what knowledge is produced and how that knowledge is produced.

With industrial societies becoming more complex, Althusser emphasised the increasing significance of such institutions in imposing capitalistic ideology on the working classes, referring to them as ideological state apparatuses (ISAs). ISAs, he argued, were much more effective in securing the consent of the masses (Crossley 2005: 152), reproducing the goals of capitalism as normal and inevitable, or as Crossley (2005: 152) conceptualises them,

> [S]ites of practice where human subjects or agents are, in effect, shaped as compliant and willing members of (capitalist) society. That is, they are the sites of practices which form us as human agents, making us what we are and, more importantly, making us "in the image" of capitalist society.

To summarise, a Marxist ideological critique which follows the ideas of Gramsci and Althusser investigates

> the subtle "ideological hegemony" by which institutions of civil society … promulgate ideas and beliefs that support the established order … the "ideological apparatuses" that the capitalist class use to preserve state power … and the ideological features of modern science that legitimate social policy decisions made by "experts" in the interests of the dominant class. (Waitzkin 1978: 270)

Effectively, hegemony functions to pacify revolutionary protest through making certain limited concessions to the working classes (e.g., by introducing and extending parliamentary democracy), while the ISAs become increasingly important in reinforcing the norms and values of the ruling classes as a consensual and widely shared view of social reality.

Of all the areas of civil society, Habermas argued that the sciences offered the greatest potential for acting as ISAs. This was due to the rhetorical language of the sciences which promoted its various disciplines as fundamentally objective and value-free. According to Habermas, scientific ideology was increasingly working on technical solutions to social and political problems within capitalist society. In this manner, states Waitzkin (2000: 122), "science tends to depoliticize these issues by removing them from critical scrutiny." Of great pertinence to understanding psychiatric discourse as hegemonic in neoliberal society, Habermas (cited in Waitzkin 2000: 122) was already claiming in 1971 that, "today's dominant, rather glassy background ideology, which makes a fetish of science, is more irresistible and far-reaching than ideologies of the old type." Increasingly, the different branches of science are responsible for legitimating fundamental inequalities in advanced capitalist societies as "normal," "inevitable," and "natural." For example, Navarro (1986: 40–41, emphasis original) states of the health system that it serves "a very high legitimization function" for capital in this regard,

> [I]t creates false consciousness that what is basically a collective and, therefore, political problem, determined by the manner of control over the process of production and consumption in capitalist societies, can be solved by individual therapeutic intervention. In this way, medicine depoliticizes what is intrinsically a political problem. Thus, what requires a collective answer is presented as an individual problem, demanding an individual response. This is a main ideological function of medicine, the *legitimization* of class relations in our society.

There are a number of specific interventions relevant to psychiatric practice which Waitzkin (2000: 124) has detailed as part of this legitimation process—these include the increasing medicalisation of social problems, "the transmission of ideological messages" within professional–client interactions, "the management of potentially troublesome emotions" by the discipline, and the reproduction of the "class structure and the relations of capitalist production." Following Freidson's (1988) work on medical dominance, Waitzkin (2000: 123) hypothesises that

> doctors may be more effective in enforcing societal norms than other social control agents; doctors are less accountable to the public and therefore freer to inject class and professional biases into their relationships with clients. Medical social control thus has extended to economic production, the family and other major institutions.

As a part of this medical social control, how and why the psychiatric discourse has become hegemonic within neoliberal society will be discussed in the following sections.

The "Public Language" of the DSM-III

Speaking at the annual meeting of the American Psychiatric Association in 1965, Mike Gorman (at the time, executive director of the National Committee Against Mental Illness) called for the psychiatric profession to develop new skills, procedures, and practices to confront the challenges posed by deinstitutionalisation and the mounting critics of the current mental health system (Chap. 1). Fundamentally, psychiatry was not speaking to the people. The middle class "worried well" spent years in private therapy hoping to learn what was really going in their unconscious, while the working classes still faced a largely coercive system of public psychiatry in institutions or outpatient facilities. It was time, Gorman argued, for psychiatry to justify itself to an increasingly cynical public who often felt that whatever "mental illness" was, it was someone else's problem. Reflecting the disenchantment of many within the APA, Gorman (cited in Harris 1995: xv, emphasis added) stated that

> *psychiatry must develop a "public" language, decontaminated of technical jargon and suited to the discussion of universal problems of our society* ... As difficult as this task is, it must be done if psychiatry is to be heard in the civic halls of our nation.

Fast-forward 50 years and it is clear that the profession has succeeded in this aim, so much so that we now often articulate the behaviour and emotions of ourselves and others using the "public language" that the psy-professionals have honed over this period. Generally, when we make assessments of character, we are now reiterating the dominant psychiatric code—for example, "your kid's a bit hyperactive," "those guys in the IT department are all on the [autistic] spectrum," "she's obviously experiencing mental health issues today," "I've just got a compulsive personality," "he's totally addicted to gaming," "you sound clinically depressed," and so on. It is perhaps hard to remember that it was not always like this. Before the 1980s a different language was used to articulate our feelings and emotions—we were perhaps "down" or sad sometimes, overjoyed or elated at other times, but seldom "manic," "clinically depressed," or indeed "bipolar." As Furedi (2004: 84) similarly notes of the rise of "therapeutic culture" in the west, "[b]efore the 1980s, terms like syndrome, self-esteem, PTSD, sex addiction and counselling had not yet entered the public vocabulary." And few desired access to labels of mental disorder either (which, at the time, involved a high risk of being hospitalised). When mental illnesses were identified in public discourse, it was typically limited to highly stigmatised categories such as schizophrenia or manic-depression. This has obviously changed. Here I locate the fundamental reason for this as due to the decline of social welfarism and the rise of neoliberalism in the 1970s; this change facilitates the expansion of the psy-disciplines into many new areas of social and economic life. The institution of psychiatry emerges as an ISA because the psychiatric discourse becomes increasingly important in reinforcing the dominant goals of neoliberalism, focusing on the self—rather than the group, community, organisation, or society—as the appropriate site for change and (using the language of neoliberalism) "growth."

As was outlined in Chap. 1, western psychiatry was in a state of professional and epistemological crisis in the 1970s (see, e.g., Decker 2007; Mayes and Horwitz 2005; Wilson 1993), a situation which was only averted with the publication of the DSM-III in 1980. Despite the failure to in any way improve the actual "science" of psychiatry, the hype that the DSM-III task force and the APA leadership created around the manual as scientifically more rigorous than ever before worked as an excellent public relations exercise for the profession. The DSM-III was also a decisive victory for biomedical psychiatry, a return to the descriptive "scientific psychiatry" of the early twentieth century. Thus, the DSM-III can also be seen as an attempt at internal legitimation, to align their activities and practices more closely to other branches of medicine. As a result of this return to biomedicine, the DSM-III was primarily promoting drug solutions to the mental disorders catalogued therein, a situation that has led many commentators to highlight the strong financial linkage between task force members and pharmaceutical companies (see, e.g., Cosgrove and Wheeler 2013). The rapid growth in the total number of mental disorders from DSM-II to DSM-III (from 182 to 265, the largest single expansion to date) also suggested a move by psychiatry to increasingly (bio)medicalise aspects of life which had previously fallen outside of the profession's domain, a process to further expand their areas of jurisdiction.

Due to the success of the DSM-III, Samson (1995: 79) states that the manual has become "the most important source of professional legitimation worldwide," and one which has had serious consequences outside of psychiatry itself. As Mayes and Horwitz (2005: 265) have since summarised of the effects of the DSM-III,

> The direct and indirect institutional change the new manual produced extended far beyond psychiatry, because the DSM is used by clinicians, the courts, researchers, insurance companies, managed care organizations, and the government (NIMH, FDA, Medicaid, Medicare). As a classificatory scheme, it categorizes people as normal or disabled, healthy or sick. And as the definitive manual for measuring and defining illness and disorders, it operates as mental health care's official language for clinical research, financial reimbursement, and professional expertise. Few professional documents compare to the DSM in terms of affecting the welfare of so many people.

While critical assessments of the DSM-III which expose the document as an important example of professional retrenchment and jurisdictional expansion—in other words, a fundamentally political rather than scientific project (Armstrong, in Caplan 1995: ix)—have validity, not enough attention has been paid to the wider societal processes effecting the institution during the period when the DSM-III was constructed and produced (in fact, neo-Foucauldian scholars such as Nikolas Rose

(1996, 1999) are probably the only ones to make the connection between the emerging "advanced liberal" conditions and the expansion of psy-discourse and services). In the 1970s, western society is in a period of serious social and economic upheaval. These issues cannot be separated from the crisis within psychiatry in the 1970s, nor the solution offered by the DSM-III in 1980. Instead, the development of the DSM-III can be better understood as a part of the structural changes informed by the decline of the social state and the emergence of neoliberal ideology.

Fundamentally, the DSM-III began to speak the "public language" that Gorman had advocated 15 years earlier. Such adaptation of professional knowledge to more consumer-friendly terminology was not unique to psychiatry but witnessed across a range of professions. For instance, Oppenheimer made the observation in the mid-1970s that professionals were increasing called upon "to systematize their knowledge and thereby make it potentially accessible to lay members of society" (Macdonald 1995: 4). Whereas the DSM-I and the DSM-II were primarily developed for use by doctors in the hospital system, Decker (2013: xvii, emphasises added) explains that the DSM-III "was meant instead for psychiatrists in private practice, *mainly seeing patients one to one*, and for research psychiatrists in academic institutions, *carrying out a host of studies on many patients at a time.*" Consequently, the language and phrasing of mental disorders in the DSM-III was simplified and made more intelligible to the lay community. For consultations with clients and for research (e.g., the increasing use of mass-survey data collection, which developed with the DSM-III field trials and continues today), simple articulations as opposed to jargon-laden typologies of disease were required. The DSM-III offered an example of Althusser's (2005) concept of "interpellation"—people began to recognise their own behaviour in the descriptions of mental pathology in the manual, lists of "symptoms" that could be easily utilised in quantifiable researcher checklists as well as self-report studies which encouraged people to begin diagnosing themselves with such disorders. For the first time, each disorder in the DSM-III was presented with a handy list of specific diagnostic criteria, which spoke simultaneously to everyone as well as in such a vague manner as to facilitate the stretching of the psychiatric net much wider than before. For instance, the diagnostic criteria for overanxious disorder included "unrealistic worry about future events," "preoccupation with the appropriateness of the individual's behaviour in the past," "overconcern about competence in a variety of areas," "excessive need for reassurance about a variety of worries," "marked self-consciousness or susceptibility to embarrassment or humiliation," and "marked feelings of tension or inability to relax" (American Psychiatric Association, 1980: 56–57).

More generally, however, the psychiatric discourse witnessed in the DSM-III (as well as subsequent DSMs) reflects the emergence of neoliberal obsessions with efficiency, productivity, and consumption (Chaps. 4–7). So when we conceptualise psychiatry as speaking a "public language" in the DSM, it must be recognised that this language is not neutral and value-free but rather reflects a dominant ideological rhetoric of the specific epoch, in this case the crisis in welfarism and the emergence of neoliberalism. The priorities and proclivities of western psychiatry cannot be seen as motivated primarily by professional interest or by economic motives of the pharmaceutical industry but instead as framed by prevailing norms and values of the social order. As a political document, the discourse articulated in the DSM-III reflects the changing nature of late capitalism. Table 3.1 gives a straightforward example of this, highlighting the increased use of phrasings attached to work, home, and school with each edition of the DSM. Whereas the DSM-I and the DSM-II make hardly any reference to such arenas of life, the DSM-III dramatically increases such phrasing—a trend which continues as neoliberalism progresses. It is also interesting to note that there was a significant increase in the use of the "work" and "school" phrasings between the DSM-IV-TR (in 2000) and the DSM-5 (in 2013), despite the manuals being of almost equal length.

Table 3.1 Increase in the use of work, home, and school phrasings in the DSM, 1952–2013[a]

Word/phrase	DSM-I (1952)	DSM-II (1968)	DSM-III (1980)	DSM-III-R (1987)	DSM-IV (1994)	DSM-IV-TR (2000)	DSM-5 (2013)
Work/ing/er	5	1	72	122	186	204	288
Home/housework	2	2	59	80	92	96	109
School	4	2	91	105	158	170	257

[a]See Appendix A for methodology

Like every profession, psychiatry has a degree of autonomy in their research and practices, yet they are ultimately shaped by current power relations. The priorities of the profession, therefore, tend to mirror the priorities of capitalism. To illustrate this point with another example, Lane (2007) has profiled how shyness became the new mental disorder of social phobia (since relabelled as social anxiety disorder) in the DSM-III (Chap. 4). With no validity for such a diagnosis, a number of parties are implicated in this case of medicalisation including the Pfizer pharmaceutical corporation (who funded a number of task force meetings at the time) and Robert Spitzer's fight with the psychoanalysts for control of diagnostic constructions. However, these issues are predated by the profession's own research focus on shyness which can be traced back to the mid-1960s, with a small number of patients showing symptoms of anxiety around social situations such as visiting the office canteen, attending parties, or being involved in public speaking (Lane 2007: 71). As would progress further under the neoliberalist doctrine, the development of new classifications such as social phobia would appear to the profession to originate in some sort of "evidence base" (which are actually people's problems in adjusting to changing arrangements of capital in arenas such as work, home, and the school). Psychiatry then does in fact maintain a key role in setting the agenda for what potentially ends up in the DSM; however, the origins of that agenda are external to the profession, dictated by wider social and economic forces. By the time of the DSM-5, psychiatric diagnoses are blatantly mirroring neoliberal ideology in relating mental illness to underperformance. With the diagnostic criteria for premenstrual dysphoric disorder (PMDD), for example, the manual (American Psychiatric Association 2013: 172, emphasis added) states that "[t]he symptoms are associated with clinically significant distress or interference with work, school, usual social activities, or relationships with others (e.g., avoidance of social activities; *decreased productivity and efficiency* at work, school, or home)." Thus, the prevailing ideological values of our time—for instance, to be productive and efficient in all aspects of our lives—is conceived through psychiatric discourse as a common sense mental health message. Are you failing within neoliberal society? Then you might have a mental illness. As Conrad and Potter (2000: 561–562) have summated of psychiatry's diagnostic project here, the process is necessarily historically and culturally contingent: "[c]ertain diagnostic categories appear and disappear over time, reflecting and reinforcing particular ideologies within the 'diagnostic project' (the professional legitimization of diagnoses), as well as within the larger social order."

Beginning with the success of the DSM-III, this section has mapped how the psychiatric discourse reflects and reproduces the dominant ideology of late capitalism. The reason for its progression to a state of hegemonic authority on the self requires discussion of the main tenets of neoliberal philosophy. These will be examined in the following section.

The Rise of Neoliberalism and Hegemonic Psychiatry

The post-war period of social welfarism and popular state intervention in many spheres of social and economic activity (including state provision of health and welfare services, public housing, nationalised industries, and a highly regulated labour market) effectively came to an end in the 1970s with high levels of inflation and unemployment (conceptualised by contemporary commentators as "stagflation") (Schrecker and Bambra 2015: 13). In this climate there was a popular response from the economic elites—and then the electorates—to the "neoliberal" ideas of economic philosophers such as Hayek (1976) and Friedman (1982) who argued that the well-being of the individual was predicated on the autonomy and freedom of the market in capitalist societies. According to these commentators, the crisis in contemporary economic and social conditions was due to the over-regulation and control of the market by the state. Centralised planning and over-bureaucratisation of the marketplace had been a detriment to the competition and potential growth of western economies (Rose 1996: 153). Under such conditions, neoliberal thinkers argued that individuals could not reach their full potential, achieve substantial success, and consequently maximise their own happiness. Neoliberal philosophy then framed old laissez faire economic arguments in a new conception of personal emancipation; it appeared simultaneously as a "pragmatic" response to changing global processes and as a popular "freeing" of the people from the constraints of central governments. As Harvey (2005: 40) has noted of this selling of the neoliberal project to the masses,

> An open project around the restoration of economic power to a small elite would probably not gain much popular support. But a programmatic attempt to advance the cause of individual freedoms could appeal to a mass base and so disguise the drive to restore class power. Furthermore, once the state apparatus made the neoliberal turn it could use its powers of persuasion, co-optation, bribery, and threat to maintain the climate of consent necessary to perpetuate its power.

Schrecker and Bambra (2015: 13) have commented that neoliberalism can be best understood as having multiple dimensions, "including concrete policy programs and innovations (e.g., welfare state retrenchment and 'workfare'), more general reorganization of state institutions (e.g., privatization and contracting out), and an ideology." In the first instance, neoliberalism is an economic theory which seeks to free capital from government regulation and restraint in the belief that this is the most successful and efficient means of achieving wealth and happiness for the greatest number. Or as Harvey (2005: 2) states of the idea, it proposes "that human well-being can best be advanced by liberating individual entrepreneurial freedoms and skills within an institutional framework characterized by strong private property rights, free markets, and free trade." The popularity of this political philosophy crystallised in the late 1970s with the electoral successes of the Thatcher and Reagan governments in the United Kingdom and United States, respectively. Backed by international financial institutions such as the International Monetary Fund and the World Bank, "liberalisation" policies were quickly introduced which "freed" local markets from state interference and saw a massive redistribution of resources from the public to the private sector, including the selling-off of state industries and assets (Moncrieff 2008: 237–238). At the same time, these neoconservative governments cut public spending in such areas as health, housing, education, social services, and welfare.

As devastating as the neoliberal economic policies of the 1970s and 1980s were to the working classes, it was the ideological aspects of the philosophy which had the greater and longer lasting impact on western society. In Moncrieff's (2008: 241) words, what accompanied the economic polices was "an evolving cultural and moral ethos, which is best summed up by a change from broad acceptance of collective virtues such as equality and solidarity to the individual and intertwined values of competition and consumerism." As with the "freeing" of capital from state intervention, neoliberal philosophy argued that the individual must also be "freed" from the state. To "aid" or "encourage" the individual to be competitive and maximise their potential within this society, neoliberal governments made radical cuts in spending on social services and welfare provision, instead channelling resources into training and workfare programmes, nominally aimed at encouraging entrepreneurship and proactive citizens into employment and business opportunities. Fundamentally, this brought about a seismic shift in the popular perception of the state from being a provider of care and services to the population to one aimed at facilitating (both market and individual) competition. The move from "welfare capitalism" to "workfare capitalism" has been summated by Schrecker and Bambra (2015: 16) as a move to "decentralization and welfare pluralism (with a strong role for the private sector), the promotion of labour market flexibility, supply-side economics, the subordination of social policy to the demands of the market and a desire to minimize social expenditure."

The withdrawal of the state from many areas of social and community activity and the refocusing instead on the individual as the site of responsibility and transformation begins to explain how the psy-disciplines came to expand their areas of jurisdiction with neoliberalism. Rose (1996: 150–151) eloquently refers to the populace in this new set of political and social relations as "enterprising individuals," that is, subjects embedded with the core values of neoliberalism. This includes the very language we now use to speak of and understand ourselves—as autonomous individuals seemingly free to choose, yet personally responsible for non-achievement. As Harvey (2005: 65–66) suggests of the neoliberal self,

> While personal and individual freedom in the marketplace is guaranteed, each individual is held responsible and accountable for his or her own actions and well-being … Individual success or failure are interpreted in

> terms of entrepreneurial virtues or personal failings (such as not investing significantly enough in one's own human capital through education) rather than being attributed to any systemic property (such as the class exclusions usually attributed to capitalism).

Popular consent for such a conception of the self has been achieved through "[p]owerful ideological influences circulated through the corporations, the media, and the numerous institutions that constitute civil society—such as the universities, schools, churches, and professional associations" (Harvey 2005: 40). Here we can obviously add the psy-professions as a part of civil society responsible for promoting such neoliberal values. Harvey (2005: 3) concludes that neoliberalism "as a mode of discourse" has become hegemonic. How we understand ourselves and the world is both shaped by and relies on the dominant language of the "enterprise culture." In other words, the discourse traditionally associated with business and economics (e.g., "efficiency," "productivity," and so on) is now also used to refer to our own experiences, emotions, and behaviour. In neoliberal ideology, the self has replaced the group, the community, or wider society as the site for reform and change. This emphasis on the individual has seen the depoliticisation of social and economic inequalities to the point where, in the words of Ulrich Beck (1992: 100, emphasis original), they have been redefined "in terms of an *individualization of social risks.*" Most pertinent to our understanding of the psy-professions in neoliberal society is that "social problems are increasingly perceived in terms of psychological dispositions: as personal inadequacies, guilt feelings, anxieties, conflicts, and neuroses" (Beck 1992: 100). In this "risk society," "expert" groups such as psychiatrists and psychologists become increasingly important to capitalism in their attempts to scientifically speak to the "risky" behaviour of the individual. This rise of "expert knowledge and expert opinion" in neoliberal society, remarks Turner (1995: 221), means that such discourse is "highly politicized." Thus, as the social state has fallen away with the expansion of neoliberal ideology, the psy-disciplines have come to play a key role in promoting and perpetuating the focus on the risky subject, increasing their moral authority into new areas of jurisdiction, with every individual within a population redefined under a hegemonic psychiatric discourse as "in a permanent condition of vulnerability" (Furedi 2004: 130) to "mental illness."

Through an understanding of the rise of neoliberalism, it is therefore possible to comprehend the recent expansion of the psychiatric discourse. For Rose (1999: vii), the psy-professions have played "a very significant role in contemporary forms of political power," so much so, that the disciplines "make it possible to govern human beings in ways that are compatible with the principles of liberalism and democracy." This is due to their professional focus on character reform and self-realization, values which have a high degree of symmetry with the neoliberal project. As has been discussed, in 1980 the DSM-III expanded the APA's range of mental disorders and made the diagnoses more user-friendly. It began to speak the language of neoliberalism, highlighting everyday issues in settings beyond the institution. Rather than only disability and illness, recovery and growth were now also promoted as possible. Moskowitz gives an example of this change in emphasis with the introduction of the diagnosis of identity disorder in the 1980s, the DSM stating that potential sufferers had

> uncertainty about a variety of issues relating to identity, including long-term goals, career choice, friendship patterns, sexual orientation, and behaviour, religious identification, moral value systems and group loyalties ... Frequently, the disturbance is epitomized by the person asking "Who am I?" (American Psychiatric Association, cited in Moskowitz 2001: 246)

Previously dominated by the negative institutional classifications of schizophrenia and manic-depression, the expanding range of personality, identity, and anxiety disorders from the DSM-III onwards has initiated a more "positive" discourse of day-to-day concerns, inadequacies, and traumas. In the post-institutional climate, acute and severe mental disorders have been replaced with the now "common disorders" of ADHD, post-traumatic stress disorder (PTSD), general anxiety disorder, BPD, and autism, for which the prescribed treatment is much more likely to be drugs or therapy rather than committal. The impressive results of this neoliberal shift in the psychiatric discourse towards the idea of "positive" mental health can be seen in the countless "awareness campaigns" invoking the risk of mental illness within the general population ("it's everyone's problem"), as well as the mass screenings and "early intervention" programmes in schools to "catch" the early phases of mental illness in children and thereby "prevent" a more serious disorder in adulthood. Further examples include the expanding number of epidemiological studies which claim to highlight yet more cases of mental pathology which have gone undetected and/or untreated in the community, the grassroots movements campaigning for further aspects of behaviour or personality to also be classified as an official mental disorder, and the general high levels of self-labelling within the population.

Similarly, it is more than coincidence that the 1980s and 1990s saw the rise of self-help culture (Ehrenreich 2009; Moskowitz 2001) and the turn of psychological and counselling professionals towards "positive psychology" and "positive thinking" (Cederström and Spicer 2015: 62–63). Laid thick with the values of neoliberalism, the discourse of "positive mental health" no longer focuses primarily on bringing the "insane" back to some state of normality but rather on the self-improvement of the individual. It is no longer enough to be "sane" or "normal"; one has to be constantly striving to be more positive and happier in life. This is a therapeutic quest which perfectly aligns with the neoliberal philosophy of personal responsibility and the need to constantly improve the self. It is a hegemonic discourse, thinly veiled as a therapeutic and medical expertise on the mind which promotes the values and goals of neoliberal capital. As Ehrenreich (2009: 8–9) has stated of the "positive thinking" revolution in late capitalism, it promotes a model of deficit focused entirely on the individual:

> If optimism is the key to material success, and if you can achieve an optimistic outlook through the discipline of positive thinking, then there is no excuse for failure. The flip side of positivity is thus a harsh insistence on personal responsibility: if your business fails or your job is eliminated, it must [be] because you didn't try hard enough, didn't believe firmly enough in the inevitability of your success. As the economy has brought more layoffs and financial turbulence to the middle class, the promoters of positive thinking have increasingly emphasized this negative judgment: to be disappointed, resentful, or downcast is to be a "victim" and a "whiner."

In the same way, psychiatric labels have come to focus on deficits and failings in character which threaten the productivity and consumption activities of the individual in many social and economic arenas of life. Thus, the psychiatric discourse seeks to both depoliticise the fundamental inequalities and structural failings of capitalism as individual coping problems while reinforcing the values of competition and self-improvement as common sense and taken for granted. Speaking similarly of psychotherapy, Parker (2014: 171) states that the individual's

> "adaptation" to capitalism requires psychotherapists not merely to ameliorate the worst excesses of the system, but to ensure that this adaptation is geared to inciting and channelling the critical reflexive energy of citizens so that the very critique that they make of the economy serves to fine-tune it … Thus psychotherapy becomes crucial to the state health apparatus as a practice devoted to the balance of dissatisfaction and yearning requisite for consumption and production.

To explain more fully how we have come to self-regulate ourselves under a hegemonic psychiatric discourse in neoliberal society, the next section draws on Foucault's theory of bio-power, a subtle form of regulatory power focused on the body.

Bio-Power, Governance, and Psychiatric Hegemony

To counter the claim that psychiatry acts as an agent of social control, such professionals commonly point to the many clients who now voluntary approach them demanding a psychiatric label (and often specify the medication which they see as the solution to their chosen disorder). They also highlight the many grassroots organisations which have sprung up to support the "reality" of various mental disorders (e.g., Autism Speaks, Children and Adults with Attention-Deficit/Hyperactivity Disorder, and the Depression and Bipolar Support Alliance) with anti-stigma campaigns and calls to "normalise" these afflictions in line with a growing disabilities discourse (Conrad 2007: 87). Further, professionals can cite the global flow of biomedical ideas on mental illness which people are increasingly communicating through social media without any direct intervention from the experts (as an example, I was recently forwarded an image from a "friend" on Facebook showing brain scans of four "normal" people and four suffering from ADHD, PTSD, bipolar disorder, and depression—cue the conclusion that different coloured blobs in the head are the cause of different mental illnesses—"just because you can't see it," read the accompanying statement, "doesn't mean someone's not battling it"). Reflecting on these acts of self-monitoring and promotion of the psychiatric discourse from the behavioural and happiness sciences, Davies (2015: 258) notes that the greatest success of such knowledge claims occurs "when individuals come to interpret and narrate their own lives according to this body of expertise."

For Foucault, the emergence of industrial society marked a transformation in the exercise of power from the right to *take life* to power *over life* (Smart 1983: 90). This was a change in the nature of sovereign power towards a focus on the biological; the body becomes an increasingly important site for the surveillance and governance of the individual. Under the developing system of production, populations are to be supervised and managed through more subtle systems of regulation and social control, with health and social services being particularly significant to the emergence and expansion of bio-power. As Smart (1983: 90) explains,

> [T]he well-being of the population or the social body was the object of techniques of power, the focus of their exercise being the conditions affecting the biological processes of life (e.g. reproduction, mortality, health, etc.). The emergence of these respective techniques for subjugating bodies and for regulating populations has been identified by Foucault as marking the beginning of an era of bio-power.

Bio-power is thus the merging of the biological with the political. Under new expert authorities in industrial society, the body becomes an object of knowledge to be monitored, coerced, and controlled in increasingly complex ways. Through these techniques the body is made "docile" so as to be "subjected, used, transformed, and improved" (Foucault, cited in Gastaldo 1997: 114). Expert forms of knowledge on the body such as those produced by the psy-professionals become increasingly important in advanced liberal societies as they can regulate individuals beyond the traditional sites of state intervention. This general process of regulation of the population beyond the direct, overt apparatus of the state has been referred to in a Foucauldian sense as modes of "governance." "Governmentality" was defined by Foucault (cited in Rose et al. 2006: 83) as "techniques and procedures for directing human behaviour." In Rose's (1996: 155, emphasis original) words,

> Governing in a liberal-democratic way means governing *through* the freedom and aspirations of subjects rather than in spite of them. The possibility of imposing "liberal" limits on the extent and scope of "political" rule has thus been provided by a proliferation of discourses, practices, and techniques through which self-governing capabilities can be installed in free individuals in order to bring their own ways of conducting and evaluating themselves into alignment with political objectives.

Rose would disagree, but I believe that these political objectives are to reinforce class rule and facilitate the maximisation of profits for the elites. As the social state has declined, the governance of individuals through neoliberal health and wellness discourses—including psychiatric ideology—has allowed for a more subtle form of social control to emerge, one that governs bodies "at a distance" through the extension of bio-politics. This is the expansion of ruling class hegemony through the spread of psychiatric myths into previously untouched areas of social and economic life. It is a most profound form of social control, as it appears in daily life as if we have consented to this expansion of psychiatric authority. After all, no one forced us to recognise our own unproductiveness because we spend too much time at the computer playing solitaire; rather, we now seem to be proactive in realising we have a "problem"—anything from attention-deficit and work avoidance behaviour to gaming addiction and obsessive behaviour—and require "help." Thus, an important part of bio-politics in neoliberal society is self-surveillance, with Rose (1999: 11, emphasis added) noting that,

> Through self-inspection, self-problematization, self-monitoring, and confession, *we evaluate ourselves according to the criteria provided for us by others.* Through self-reformation, therapy, techniques of body alteration, and calculated reshaping of speech and emotion, we adjust ourselves by means of

> the techniques propounded by the experts of the soul [meaning, the psy-professionals].

For neo-Foucauldian scholars, this governance at a distance is not necessarily a negative thing. Instead, it can empower individuals in negotiating their many public and personal responsibilities, and in understanding the limits of their actions and behaviour in society. Yet at its heart, notes Furedi, this "therapeutic governance" has a weak conception of individual capacity. It remains a top-down view of the individual which "represents scepticism towards the ability of people to act as responsible citizens, without the support of professionals who knows [sic] best what is in their interest" (Furedi 2004: 196). Instead, it can be more accurately hypothesised that the current popularity of mental health self-surveillance and mental illness self-labelling results from psychiatric hegemony and its imbued neoliberal ideology of risk and personal responsivity. As Clarke et al. (2003: 171–172) have stated of this focus on medical surveillance in neoliberal society,

> [H]ealth becomes an individual goal, a social and moral responsibility, and a site for routine biomedical intervention ... the focus is no longer on illness, disability, and disease as matters of fate, but on health as a matter [of] ongoing moral self-transformation.

Through psychiatric hegemony, then, we are all implicated as "at risk" of mental illness and must constantly self-monitor for potential signs of disorder (as many professional associations and drug adverts advise us). Clarke (2013: 418) has summated the importance of this mental health self-governance in neoliberal society with reference to the rise of disorders such as ADHD. She states,

> Neo-liberal governance is typified by its emphasis on citizen involvement as individuals take independent action and become enterprises (or entrepreneurs) unto themselves and in a sense police themselves by internalising and enacting prevailing truths about the identification and management of risks ... Neo-liberalism depends on self-governance (or in the case of children, governance by parents and similar authorities). For instance, mothers increasingly turn to ... individualising children's (mis)behaviour as disordered through mental illness discourse, of which attention deficit disorder

(ADD)/Attention deficit hyperactivity disorder (ADHD) is the most prevalent around the globe today.

The parent has successfully sought help and aided the medicalisation of the child's deviant behaviour (Chap. 5). This is a neoliberal process of social control which is so successful that Norris and Lloyd (cited in Adams 2008: 119) have noticed that the mental illness diagnosis often comes as a relief to the parent

> first, because they have located the "cause" of their child's distress, and secondly, because they, as parents, are not to blame ... Their child's "abnormal" behaviour is, in this account, a medical issue to be rectified through medication that makes "normal" their child's brain dysfunction.

What is also evident here is that the biomedical model is crucial to promoting neoliberal solutions focused on the individual. This successfully depoliticises the non-conformity of the child through suggesting that "chemical imbalances" in the brain are the problem. As a frontline psychiatrist herself, Moncrieff (2008: 243) has recognised that the rise of biomedical psychiatry and neoliberalism are intrinsically linked: "the chemical imbalance idea of psychiatric problems facilitates the neoliberal project," she argues, and "features of neoliberalism in turn strengthen the chemical balance theory and biopsychiatry more generally." The increasing social and economic disparities in neoliberal society are individualised through biomedical ideology. Moncrieff (2008: 248–249) states that this represents

> a clear instance of the medicalization of political discontent. But this situation is not overtly coercive. This view has not been imposed on people by direct force. People themselves have come to see their problems as individual problems, emanating from their brain chemistry.

Thus, biomedical ideology as a part of psychiatric hegemony has become the dominant "solution" to what are social and economic conditions of late capitalism. Biomedicine promises a range of corrections in line with neoliberal conduct, such as improved productivity and marketability as well as "recovery" and the "normalisation" of mental disorders for those who are at risk of deviating from their expected roles as workers, consumers, students, homemakers, and reproducers of the future workforce. Yet psychiatric hegemony encompasses more than the dominant biomedical rhetoric, and can also be detected in social models of the psy-professions. Feminist therapists, for example, argue that a legitimate response to a climate of anti-feminism is now to work on the self-esteem of their clients. "Hence," remarks Dubrofsky (2007: 266), "social, political, and economic problems are turned into personal problems that can be solved by an individual who is willing to work on him- or herself." It is but one example of an all-encompassing psychiatric discourse that denies the social and political realities of late capitalism and has successfully placed the focus back on the individual as the site of change.

Summary

Thirty-five years ago, Ingelby (1980: 54) predicted an expansion of psychiatric ideology into the public sphere when he stated that psychiatric ideas were being "incorporated within 'common sense' itself." No longer was the mental patient to be subject to overt forms of oppression within the psychiatric institution; rather, the patient would come to embody psychiatric discourse on a more voluntary basis. "For as the mental hospitals are phased out," remarked Ingelby (1980: 54),

> more and more treatment takes place in the doctor's surgery and the general hospital; but the mental patient is still just as effectively incarcerated within his role. Moreover, this role is internalized within the patient's own thinking and that of the people around him or her, and it guides everybody's self-interpretations, whether or not they ever become patients.

As the neoliberal project has developed, we have all become implicated as subjects at risk of mental disorder. This is not, however, due to any advancement in the knowledge on real pathology but rather an expansion of the psychiatric discourse to the point where it has taken on hegemonic status. It is more than coincidence then that, as Davies (2015: 177) has observed, "[t]he entanglement of psychic maximization and profit maximization has grown more explicit over the course of the neoliberal era." As I have argued in this chapter, neoliberalism requires a compliant and competitive population focused on correcting and improving their emotions, behaviour, and social capacities. This has been aided by the expansion of the psy-professions in governing populations "at a distance"; psychiatric hegemony has depoliticised fundamental inequalities of capitalism while proliferating neoliberal values through its classifications and philosophies on "treatment." The pretext of scientific authority on the mind has allowed the psy-professions to enforce ruling class values and norms as consensual and taken-for-granted assumptions of human behaviour. This has happened to such an extent that individuals are now involved in acts of self-surveillance, seeking the solution to the structural failings of neoliberal society through individual DSM symptoms of "mental illness."

The psychiatric profession has always been a site of social control for policing the working classes within industrial society, yet their ideological role has never been as significant as it currently is. Over the chapters that follow, I will systematically demonstrate the development of this psychiatric hegemony by drawing on the evidence of psy-expansionism into the world of work and employment, through exploring youth deviance and the education system, through investigating the social control of women and the reinforcement of the division of labour, and with the continued pathologisation of social and political dissent.

Bibliography

Adams, P. (2008) 'Positioning Behaviour: Attention Deficit/Hyperactivity Disorder (ADHD) in the Post-Welfare Educational Era', *International Journal of Inclusive Education*, 12(2): 113–125.

Althusser, L. (2005) *For Marx*. London: Verso.

American Psychiatric Association. (1980) *Diagnostic and Statistical Manual of Mental Disorders* (3rd ed.). Washington, DC: American Psychiatric Association.

American Psychiatric Association. (2013) *Diagnostic and Statistical Manual of Mental Disorders* (5th ed.). Arlington, VA: American Psychiatric Association.

Beck, U. (1992) *Risk Society: Towards a New Modernity*. London: Sage.
Caplan, P. J. (1995) *They Say You're Crazy: How the World's Most Powerful Psychiatrists Decide Who's Normal*. Cambridge, MA: De Capo Press.
Cederström, C., and Spicer, A. (2015) *The Wellness Syndrome*. Cambridge: Polity Press.
Clarke, A. E., Shim, J. K., Mamo, L., Fosket, J. R., and Fishman, J. R. (2003) 'Biomedicalization: Technoscientific Transformations of Health, Illness, and U.S. Biomedicine', *American Sociological Review*, 68(2): 161–194.
Clarke, J. N. (2013) 'Medicalisation and Changes in Advice to Mothers about Children's Mental Health Issues 1970 to 1990 as Compared to 1991 to 2010: Evidence from Chatelaine Magazine', *Health, Risk & Society*, 15(5): 416–431.
Conrad, P. (2007) *The Medicalization of Society: On the Transformation of Human Conditions into Treatable Disorders*. Baltimore: John Hopkins University Press.
Conrad, P., and Potter, D. (2000) 'From Hyperactive Children to ADHD Adults: Observations on the Expansion of Medical Categories', *Social Problems*, 47(4): 559–582.
Cosgrove, L., and Wheeler, E. E. (2013) 'Industry's Colonization of Psychiatry: Ethical and Practical Implications of Financial Conflicts of Interest in the DSM-5', *Feminism & Psychology*, 23(1): 93–106.
Crossley, N. (2005) *Key Concepts in Critical Social Theory*. London: Sage.
Davies, W. (2015) *The Happiness Industry: How the Government and Big Business Sold Us Well-Being*. London: Verso.
Decker, H. S. (2007) 'How Kraepelinian was Kraepelin? How Kraepelinian are the Neo-Kraepelinians?—From Emil Kraepelin to *DSM-III*', *History of Psychiatry*, 18(3): 337–360.
Decker, H. S. (2013) *The Making of DSM-III: A Diagnostic Manual's Conquest of American Psychiatry*. Oxford: Oxford University Press.
Dubrofsky, R. E. (2007) 'Therapeutics of the Self: Surveillance in the Service of the Therapeutic', *Television & New Media*, 8(4): 263–284.
Ehrenreich, B. (2009) *Smile or Die: How Positive Thinking Fooled America and the World*. London: Granta Publications.
Femia, J. V. (1981) *Gramsci's Political Thought: Hegemony, Consciousness, and the Revolutionary Process*. Oxford: Clarendon Press.
Fontana, B. (1993) *Hegemony and Power: On the Relation between Gramsci and Machiavelli*. Minneapolis: University of Minneapolis Press.
Freidson, E. (1988) *Profession of Medicine: A Study of the Sociology of Applied Knowledge*. Chicago: University of Chicago Press.

Friedman, M. (1982) *Capitalism and Freedom*. Chicago: University of Chicago.

Furedi, F. (2004) *Therapy Culture: Cultivating Vulnerability in an Uncertain Age*. London: Routledge.

Gastaldo, D. (1997) 'Is Health Education Good for You? Re-Thinking Health Education Through the Concept of Bio-Power', in Petersen, A., and Bunton, R. (Eds.), *Foucault, Health and Medicine* (pp. 113–133). London: Routledge.

Gramsci, A. (1971) *Selections from the Prison Notebooks*. New York: International.

Harris, T. A. (1995) *I'm OK-You're OK*. London: Arrow Books.

Harvey, D. (2005) *A Brief History of Neoliberalism*. Oxford: Oxford University Press.

Hayek, F. A. (1976) *The Constitution of Liberty*. London: Routledge and Kegan Paul.

Heiner, R. (2006) *Social Problems: An Introduction to Critical Constructivism* (2nd ed.). New York: Oxford University Press.

Ingelby, D. (1980) 'Understanding "Mental Illness"', in Ingelby, D. (Ed.), *Critical Psychiatry: The Politics of Mental Health* (pp. 23–71). New York: Pantheon Books.

Kellner, D. (2005) 'Western Marxism', in Harrington, A. (Ed.), *Modern Social Theory: An Introduction* (pp. 154–174). Oxford: Oxford University Press.

Lane, C. (2007) *Shyness: How Normal Behavior Became a Sickness*. New Haven: Yale University Press.

Macdonald, K. M. (1995) *The Sociology of Professions*. London: Sage.

Marx, K. (1971) *A Contribution to the Critique of Political Economy*. New York: International.

Marx, K., and Engels, F. (1965) *Manifesto of the Communist Party*. Beijing: Foreign Languages Press.

Mayes, R., and Horwitz, A. V. (2005) 'DSM-III and the Revolution in the Classification of Mental Illness', *Journal of the History of the Behavioral Sciences*, 41(3): 249–267.

Moncrieff, J. (2008) 'Neoliberalism and Biopsychiatry: A Marriage of Convenience', in Cohen, C. I., and Timimi, S. (Eds.), *Liberatory Psychiatry: Philosophy, Politics, and Mental Health* (pp. 235–255). Cambridge: Cambridge University Press.

Moskowitz, E.S. (2001) *In Therapy We Trust: American's Obsession with Self-Fulfillment*. Baltimore: John Hopkins University Press.

Navarro, V. (1980) 'Work, Ideology and Science: The Case of Medicine', *Social Science and Medicine*, 14(3): 191–205.

Navarro, V. (1986) *Crisis, Health, and Medicine: A Social Critique*. New York: Tavistock Publications.

Navarro, V. (1989) 'Radicalism, Marxism and Medicine', *Medical Anthropology: Cross Cultural Studies in Health and Illness*, 11(2): 195–219.

Parker, I. (2014) 'Psychotherapy under Capitalism: The Production, Circulation and Management of Value and Subjectivity', *Psychotherapy and Politics International*, 13(3): 166–175.

Rose, N. (1996) *Inventing Our Selves: Psychology, Power, and Personhood*. Cambridge: Cambridge University Press.

Rose, N. (1999) *Governing the Soul: The Shaping of the Private Self* (2nd ed.). London: Free Association Books.

Rose, N., O'Malley, P., and Valverde, M. (2006) 'Governmentality', *Annual Review of Law and Social Science*, 2: 83–104.

Samson, C. (1995) 'The Fracturing of Medical Dominance in British Psychiatry?', *Sociology of Health and Illness*, 17(2): 245–268.

Schrecker, T., and Bambra, C. (2015) *How Politics Makes Us Sick: Neoliberal Epidemics*. Houndmills, Basingstoke: Palgrave Macmillan.

Smart, B. (1983) *Foucault, Marxism and Critique*. London: Routledge & Kegan Paul.

Turner, B. S. (1995) *Medical Power and Social Knowledge* (2nd ed.). London: Sage.

Waitzkin, H. (1978) 'A Marxist View of Medical Care', *Annals of Internal Medicine*, 89(2): 264–278.

Waitzkin, H. (2000) *The Second Sickness: Contradictions of Capitalist Health Care* (rev. ed.). Lanham: Rowan & Littlefield Publishers.

Whitaker, R. (2010a) *Anatomy of an Epidemic: Magic Bullets, Psychiatric Drugs, and the Astonishing Rise of Mental Illness in America*. New York: Crown Publishers.

Williams, R. (1977) *Marxism and Literature*. Oxford: Oxford University Press.

Wilson, M. (1993) DSM-III and the Transformation of American Psychiatry: A History', *American Journal of Psychiatry*, 150(3): 399–410.

4

Work: Enforcing Compliance

In this chapter, I profile the increasing encroachment of psychiatry and the psychological sciences upon the world of work. I argue that such expansionism has served a number of key goals for the profession and for capitalism, including professional legitimation and the expansion of expertise, increased profit and the consumption of goods and services and, most importantly, the naturalisation of unequal and exploitative relations in the workplace. I will demonstrate here that it is more than coincidence that the conceptualisation of work as a form of treatment or "therapy" by psychiatrists coincided with the development of industrial capitalism in the nineteenth century. "Work therapy" continues today, yet I will show that psychiatry's role has moved from that of the social control and punishment of the unemployed and the non-able bodied in the asylums to a more subtle focus on reinforcing compliant work regimes and permanent "self-growth" ideologies on the precarious worker in neoliberal society. This exploration of dominant notions of work and unemployment therefore gives special attention to the emerging hegemonic role played by the mental health experts within the neoliberal workplace. This can be demonstrated through changes within professional practices and the psychiatric discourse embedded in the categories of "mental illness" given

B.M.Z. Cohen, *Psychiatric Hegemony*,
DOI 10.1057/978-1-137-46051-6_4

in successive DSMs since 1980. The discussion will show that psychiatry and allied psychological sciences have expanded their areas of jurisdiction into the workplace of the white-collar worker at the behest of capitalist enterprise, where self-surveillance and a continual working on the self has become a part of the increased need for an efficient, flexible, and mobile labour force.

Psychiatry has always been a conservative vocation which seeks to reinforce and maintain the status quo, where the dominant norms and values of society are normalised and deviations from them are pathologised. This is clearly evidenced when exploring psychiatric interventions in the world of work. The nature of work has changed dramatically over the last two centuries with the relations of production having grown increasingly complex; the serfs have been emancipated and replaced by an increasingly flexible and precarious pool of labour required for global growth. At the same time, what has not changed is the intervention of the psychiatric discourse to justify oppressive labour relations as normal and inevitable through the depoliticising and individualising of economic hardships in the workplace. To take but one example, I woke up one afternoon recently to find that the 2014 Noble Prize winners in psychology were suggesting that my tendency to stay up late rather than get up early was a sign of "Machiavellianism, secondary psychopathy, and exploitive narcissism" (Jonason et al. 2013: 538). Obviously, some of psychiatry's little helpers had been getting up very early in the morning to grapple with the theories of evolutionary psychology and the problem of vampires. The authors did at least admit that a limitation of their study could be the predominance of students in their sample; "night-time preferences may be strongest in college-students," state Jonason et al. (2013: 540), "because of the freedom afforded to stay up late and lessened need to work relative to adults." Behind the wackiness of such research lies a serious moral message informed by the needs of liberal democratic societies for good citizens and workers to rise early and go to bed at a reasonable time. A point summarised more generally by Phil Brown (1974: 47–48) when he states that "[a]s guardians of morality, the psychiatric-psychological establishment must put into the textbooks the definitions of mental illness that best reflect the dominant social values of the bourgeoisie."

Moral Treatment and the Work Ethic

As was discussed in Chap. 2, crucial to the early formation of the asylum attendants—later to be renamed as "alienists" and then "psychiatrists"—as a legitimate group to manage the insane was the appropriation of the "humanist" philosophy of "moral treatment" from Pinel and Tuke. In line with the dominant values of early industrial society, the exposure to and reinforcement of appropriate behaviour could correct deviant character. In theory, the "mad" would no longer be chained, tortured, and warehoused by society, instead they would be taught how to behave and act appropriately without fear of punishment. In turn, good behaviour would be rewarded with humane care and the potential to re-join the world outside the institution. The stick had been replaced by the carrot; as long as the patient could learn the rules and behaviour of this new society, they had nothing to fear.

As with the prison and workhouse, one of the primary features of moral treatment at the York Retreat was the importance of work in the daily regime of the inmates and, equally, a distain for idleness. Even if the work was of little value in itself, it reinforced a moral imperative in the mind of the deviant. As Foucault (1988a: 247) reflected,

> Work comes first in "moral treatment" as practiced at the Retreat. In itself, work possesses a constraining power superior to all forms of physical coercion, in that the regularity of the hours, the requirements of attention, the obligation to produce a result detach the sufferer from a liberty of mind that would be fatal and engage him in a system of responsibilities.

Samuel Tuke was of the opinion that "of all the modes by which patients may be induced to restrain themselves, regular employment is perhaps the most generally efficacious" (cited in Scull 1989: 90). Under such a "treatment" regime, work had a moral value in self-regulating the behaviour of the deviant. This was a new form of moral surveillance in industrial society and one which was as applicable to the prisoner, the poor, and the mad as it was to the factory worker. It is this moral authority of such management and daily regimes as found in wider capitalist society which psychiatry progressed with the expansion of institutions for the insane throughout Europe and America in the nineteenth century. The key to psychiatrists successfully establishing themselves as the "experts on the mind" was their appropriation of moral treatment as a "scientific" system of care for the management of the insane which—more that coincidentally—conformed to the values of the dominant social order. As Pollard has noted, industrial capitalism demanded "a reform of 'character' on the part of every single workman, since the previous character did not fit the new industrial system" (cited in Scull 1989: 91). A new set of competitive norms had to be taught and internalised through the new institutions by disciplinary techniques rather than coercion, and this applied as much to those labelled as "mad" as to the rest of society. Thus, the appearance and success of moral treatment can only be fully understood within the wider social and economic context in which it emerged, a point reinforced by Scull (1989: 92) when he notes,

> The insistence on the importance of the internalization of norms, the conception of how this was to be done, and even the nature of the norms that were to be internalized—in all these respects we can now see how the emerging attitude toward the insane paralleled contemporaneous shifts in the treatment of other deviants and of the normal.

Following the philosophy of moral treatment, regimes of work were established in institutions for the insane so that the chances for idleness among these deviant populations would be minimised and the work ethic could be reinforced as part of the new, dominant approach to "care." Farms were to be attached to asylums to offer the opportunity for "the kind of regular employment which greatly helped to restore men's minds" (Scull 1993: 150). However, while still stressing the therapeutic benefits of moral treatment, as the asylums grew in size, the work undertaken by patients became more orientated to the goals of the facility. Similar to prisons, inmates of asylums could be found "employed" in the asylum laundries, as farm labourers, and for undertaking other menial tasks within the institution (Scull 1993: 288–289). Thus, "work therapy" became an excuse for patients to be used as cheap labour for the smooth running of the institution. This would be a constant of inpatient existence until such establishments were phased out in the latter half of the twentieth century, with Brown (1974: 51, emphasis original) commenting on psychiatric institutions in the 1970s that

> [h]ard work, faith in one's superiors and rule-following are taught, backed up with the wide range of threats available to hospital staff. Everything done *to* the patients is seen as something *for* the patients—"work therapy," "recreational therapy," etc. Thus cheap labor on the wards and in "occupational therapy" is obtained in the guise of help.

The "Humanisation" of Work

The impact of the psychological sciences on the work environment outside the institution was not felt until after World War II. The post-war economic boom created an environment of labour shortages and low retention, and under these circumstances economic elites became increasingly interested in the "psychology" of the "productive worker." "Business managers, beset by high rates of absenteeism and job turnover," reiterates Napoli (cited in Cautin et al. 2013: 43) of the situation in America,

> took unprecedented interest in hiring the right worker and keeping him contented on the job. Management turned to psychologists ... and the amount of psychological testing quickly increased. Surveys show that in 1939 only 14 % of businesses were using such tests; in 1947 the proportion rose to 50 %, and in 1952, 75 %.

From finding and retaining the "right worker" through psychological testing developed the associated idea of the "happy worker"—an employee who, through positive reinforcements, could increase rates of productivity and, consequently, profits. Work was no longer seen only as a necessity for survival within capitalist society but a place of improvement, importantly *a place to improve oneself.* As Rose (1999: 56) has summarised of this so-called "humanization" of work, "correctly organized, productive work itself can satisfy the worker; the activity of working itself can provide rewarding personal and social relations for those engaged in it; good work can be a means to self-fulfilment." The psychological sciences had a significant role to play in the development of new techniques for the selection, management, and improvement of the workforce (Rose 1999: 82), and the branches of occupational and industrial psychology expanded significantly during this period.

Changes in the industrial base of capitalism in the 1970s only served to expand psy-professional practice still further. As the manufacturing sector was replaced in economic significance by growth in the service industries, changing skills were required within the labour force. Traditional manual labour was declining while there was a burgeoning skills gap within white collar occupations. Thus, the labour force was put under increasing pressure to "adapt" and "upskill" to meet the needs of the changing marketplace. The new aptitudes required by employers included social skills, problem-solving skills, independent and team working, a flexible approach to work, as well as workers ready to further upskill. In the future, people would have to demonstrate high levels of "employability" within their jobs and what Elraz (2013: 810) calls a "sellable self" which will be, "associated with the constant expectation to perform, manage-impression, self-promote and 'sell' oneself as an attractive product: with no 'faults', 'weaknesses' or 'limitations', always ready to be, and do 'more'." This "new subjectivity of work" (Rose 1999: 106) has meant that the individual worker has become a key site for psy-professional intervention in neoliberal society. I experienced one example of this intervention at first-hand when I was employed at a Training and Enterprise Council in England in the early 1990s. Both employees and our unemployed "clients" were offered the chance to undertake taxpayer-funded neurolinguistic programming, a business-orientated form of neurocognitive therapy. The presence of this "training initiative" is a small demonstration of the successful creep of the psychological sciences into the work environment over this period—those to be re-skilled learnt in these sessions that the way to real, long-lasting, and personally satisfying success was to examine their own weaknesses and confront their personal barriers to achieving a job. The discourse of neurolinguistic programming fitted perfectly with the dominant notions of the sellable self, where success in employment was intrinsically tied to the self-actualisation of the person; an increasing need within neoliberal capitalism to "work on the ego of the worker" (Rose 1999: 113).

The idea of "positive thinking" and the opportunity for "personal growth" brought about by the expansion of the psy-professions into the world of work has been indoctrinated on the employed and unemployed alike. Ehrenreich (2009: 45) recounts the experience of laid-off white-collar workers as follows:

> At the networking groups, boot camps, and motivational sessions available to the unemployed, I found unanimous advice to abjure anger and "negativity" in favor of an upbeat, even grateful approach to one's immediate crisis. People who had been laid off from their jobs and were spiraling down toward poverty were told to see their condition as an "opportunity" to be embraced … [T]he promised outcome was a kind of "cure": by being positive, a person might not only feel better during his or her job search, but actually bring it to a faster, happier conclusion.

I would argue that what is taken by employers, managers, benefit officers, work counsellors, and occupational psychologists as "negative thinking" is the continued ability of people to think critically about their situation and consider it in a wider political context. This is the antithesis of the required compliant employed or unemployed citizen in neoliberal society, and the psy-professions have sought to depoliticise and individualise such thinking through their expansion of hegemonic notions of "happiness," "positive thinking," and "positive mental health." As psychotherapist Richard Brouillette (2016) recently admitted, a concentration on individual narratives by the profession means that "therapy could easily become an arm of the state, seeking to 'cure' listlessness or a reluctance to work, potentially limiting social and political awareness among those it is intended to serve."

Rose (1999: 114) has noted that a focus on positive mental health in the workplace has included management policies aimed at "richness of self, self-acceptance, growth motivation, investment in living, unified outlook on life, regulation from within, independence, and adequacy of interpersonal relations." In contrast, mental *illness* in the workplace can broadly be conceived as the opposite; for example, those who are perceived as having poor interpersonal relations, who show a lack of independence, and have "negative" personality traits which limit their "growth" potential (e.g., introversion, shyness, melancholia, and pessimism).

The current prevalence of mental illness in the labour force is estimated to be one in every four workers. The Partnership for Workplace Mental Health (2006: 6) estimates that the indirect annual costs of mental illness to American employers may be as high as $100 billion. Whereas a straight Marxist analysis would suggest that the increased alienation of workers in neoliberalism leads to greater levels of sickness including mental disorder (see, e.g., Robinson 1997; Rosenthal 2010; Rosenthal and Campbell 2016), there is a need to consider the interventions of the mental health system in the world of work as increasingly useful in ideological terms, justifying the precarious conditions that we currently work under as natural and inevitable. I argue here that mental illness designations are increasingly focused on the world of work and serve an important role in depoliticising employment relations; instead of recognising power disparities in the work environment, new and/or changing diagnostic categories of mental illness encourage workers to problematise the self rather than the organisation or wider society.

Table 4.1 shows the quantity of work-related terminology used in each edition of the DSM. The number of such phrasings has significantly increased over time, from a count of 10 in the DSM-I to 387 in the DSM-5. References to "work," "working," or "worker" are particularly evident in mental disorders from 1980 onwards and, despite being a similar sized manual to the previous edition, the DSM-5 increased the use of such phrasings by almost a third (it is worth noting that part of this increase is due to the introduction of the workplace to the previously

Table 4.1 Number of work-related words/phrases in the DSM, 1952–2013[a]

Word/phrase	DSM-I (1952)	DSM-II (1968)	DSM-III (1980)	DSM-III-R (1987)	DSM-IV (1994)	DSM-IV-TR (2000)	DSM-5 (2013)
Business	4	0	8	7	9	9	11
Unemployed/ment	1	0	6	17	31	23	46
Employed/ees/ers/ment							
Flexible/ility	0	0	0	1	7	4	14
Loss of job/employment/ job loss	0	0	8	1	9	10	16
Under/unproductive/ity	0	0	10	2	11	8	12
Work/ing/er	5	1	72	122	186	204	288
Total count	10	1	104	150	253	258	387

[a]See Appendix A for methodology.

school-defined ADHD diagnosis, a classification which Conrad (2007: 139) has referred to as representing "the medicalization of underperformance"). As expected, the DSM-III in 1980 shows a large increase in the references to workplace terminology. Following the construction of DSM-III, a number of mental illness classifications have appeared which have specifically sought to pathologise behaviour and personality traits which are seen to limit the desired skills and roles of workers in the neoliberal workplace; these include disinhibited social engagement disorder and social anxiety disorder. To illustrate my argument for the workplace as a site of psychiatric hegemony I will now outline the latter diagnosis as an appropriate case study.

Case Study: Social Anxiety Disorder

First classified in the DSM-III (American Psychiatric Association 1980: 227–228) as social phobia under the notoriously vague—yet increasingly useful—lexicon of anxiety disorders, the primary symptom of social anxiety disorder (SAD) was a "persistent, irrational fear of, and compelling desire to avoid, situations in which the individual may be exposed to scrutiny by others" (American Psychiatric Association 1980: 227). As acknowledged by Lane (2007: 72–75), the development of this diagnosis by the DSM-III committee had little to do with any scientific study on the topic and much more to do with acquiring a set of descriptive, inclusionary behavioural criteria under the watchful eyes of pharmaceutical patrons such as Upjohn. By the 1990s, social phobia was being named "the disorder of the decade" (Aho 2010: 191); this situation was significantly aided—not for the last time—by a loosening in diagnostic criteria with the deletion of the phrase "compelling desire to avoid" in the revised edition of the DSM-III (American Psychiatric Association 1987: 241). With only the mental disorders of alcohol dependence and major depressive disorder affecting more people, those who currently suffer from SAD in the United States are estimated to represent at least 13 per cent of the population (Aho 2010: 191).

If there really was originally an attempt to exclude "normal" behaviour from the criteria for SAD, this appears to have completely vanished by the time of the release of the DSM-5 (American Psychiatric Association 2013: 202), where the first symptom of the disorder is now a,

> Marked fear or anxiety about one or more social situations in which the individual is exposed to possible scrutiny by others. Examples include social interactions (e.g., having a conversation, meeting unfamiliar people), being observed (e.g., eating or drinking), and performing in front of others (e.g., giving a speech).

Readers may be reflecting on whether they have also shown similar anxieties in such social situations, arguably many of us have. Is this normal behaviour—an irritating if perhaps necessary fallibility of something which maybe makes us who we are—or is it a pathology, an illness which requires treatment? Critics have argued that the APA's invention of SAD represents the successful medicalisation of shyness, a natural human emotion (Lane 2007; Scott 2006). Thus, the diagnosis can be conceptualised as a label given to those deviating from dominant neoliberal norms of the model citizen and worker who should now be assertive, gregarious, and an aggressive go-getter. As Scott (2006: 134) saliently comments, thanks to the development of the SAD label, the psy-professionals now assert that "being shy is a barrier not only to personal relationships but also to career advancement and civil interaction with strangers, acquaintances and friends."

There are a number of key reasons that have been given by scholars for the "discovery" and expansion of SAD. These include the influence of pharmaceutical companies on such "diagnostic creep," the potential for jurisdictional expansion by psychiatrists and allied professions, and the promotion of shyness as a medical problem by advocacy groups and research institutions (see, e.g., Conrad 2007; Lane 2007; Moynihan and Cassels 2005; Scott 2006). However, while there is plenty of evidence to suggest that these factors have had a significant impact on the *expansion* of SAD throughout western society, they do not explain psychiatry's original focus on shyness towards its initial appearance in the DSM-III. Such an analysis involves a wider socio-historical analysis of psychiatry's primary function within western society. Aho (2010: 201) has been one to offer such a critique of those who forward the political economic view of medicalisation as simply, "a product of recent capitalist collusion between the pharmaceutical industry, managed care organizations … and advocates of the new DSM." Instead, he states that "before medical professionals and pharmaceutical conglomerates can profit from pathologizing certain behaviors, a web of historical meanings is already in place, working behind our backs to determine what will count as normal and abnormal" (Aho 2010: 201).

As I have outlined earlier in this book, the institution of psychiatry does not work in a vacuum, somehow above the everyday norms and values of wider society; rather, they are a profession with a particular conservative zeal for upholding the current social order through their work. When behaviour becomes unacceptable to the needs of capitalism, the profession seeks to pathologise such deviance. This process does not happen overnight but through a progression of debate, research, and movement towards a collective focus on such areas. In this case, the research on shyness from Philip Zimbardo (1977)—the former president of the American Psychological Association—is seen as key towards the development of social phobia as a category of mental illness. Significantly, his research did not suggest that shyness was a mental illness, but rather noted a concern that people with such characteristics were likely to be seriously disadvantaged as society began to change. Zimbardo (1977: 5, emphasis added) commented on the "condition,"

> Shyness is an insidious personal problem that is reaching such endemic proportions as to be justifiably called a social disease. *Trends in our society suggest it will get worse in the coming years as social forces increase our isolation, competition, and loneliness.* Unless we begin to do something soon, many of our children and grandchildren will become prisoners of their own shyness.

The traits of shyness—including timidity, mistrust of others, and a lack of self-assertion (Zimbardo 1977: 13)—were conceptualised as increasingly problematic within contemporary society and therefore a justifiable focus for psychiatric activity. This is tacit acceptance that such behaviour has not been found to be a mental disorder as a result of rigorous testing but rather is socially dictated and culturally relative; shyness becomes a "social disease" (i.e., a social deviance) in need of treatment. Thus, "the rise of social phobia," states Cottle (1999: 25),

> offers a glimpse not so much at the anatomy of a specific illness as at the still inherently subjective nature of psychiatric medicine and the cultural forces that help draw the boundary between what we are told to think of as normal and what we are told to consider pathological.

Concerned with the need for workers to conform to the desired norms and values necessary to "succeed" in neoliberal society, the psy-professions have stigmatised and "othered" those once considered only shy, introverted, or reticent co-workers. This process of psychiatrists labelling the shy as mentally ill has also been previously highlighted by Scott (2004: 133) who acknowledges that, in comparison, the non-shy self,

> embodies the cultural values of contemporary Western societies: ambition, assertiveness, competitiveness and individualism. This dominant ideal can be used to stigmatize those who fail to live up to such expectations, whose difference is attributed to individual pathologies rather than to an unrealistic cultural ideology.

The success of psychiatric hegemony here is that since the original construction of social phobia in 1980, workers have become more inclined to self-label and entertain the possibility of therapy and drug treatment for their failure to be more sociable and assertive at their place of work. This situation has further legitimated the extension of the psy-professions in the areas of unemployment, job training, and work, reinforcing the neoliberal focus on the self as the site of change, while simultaneously depoliticising the increasingly alienating work environment and constant pressures on employees to upskill and be "more employable" in the jobs market (see Elraz 2013). Through the pathologisation of such "non-sellable" traits, Lane (2007: 208) argues that what counts as acceptable behaviour within the population has been narrowed to such an extent that "we now tend to believe that active membership in community activities, the cultivation of social skills (becoming a 'people person'), and the development of group consciousness are natural, universal, and obligatory aims."

Summary

As Roberts (2015: 24) has pointed out of the recent increase in the use of the "autism" label by the psy-professions, the pathologisation of shyness reflects neoliberal capital's desire for "emotional labour" within the work force. "It is no longer enough just to shift product," states Roberts (2015: 24), "one must now do it with a smile, with 'sincerity,' with a friendly touch." In this chapter I have discussed the psy-professionals' involvement in the area of work from utilising it as a form of "therapy" for idleness in the nineteenth century to encompassing dominant neoliberal ideals of employability and productivity in the current DSM. Reinforcing the ideological prerogatives for workers to concentrate on their individual failings rather than the social reality of their collective exploitation under capitalism has allowed the experts of the mind to expand their areas of jurisdiction into the office, factory, home, and—as we shall see in the next chapter—the school.

In 2014, the Bureau of Labor Statistics ranked industrial–organisational psychologists as the fastest-growing occupation in the United States, with Farnham (2014) noting of the profession that "their expertise results in better hires, increased productivity, reduced turnover, and lower labor costs." Meanwhile, the UK government's Department for Work and Pensions has recently been considering compulsory mental health counselling for the unemployed and possible sanctions for those who refuse such "treatment" (Gayle 2015). Again we witness here the expansion of psy-professions as they align their "expertise" and "science" with the needs of capitalism. Contrary to what our managers are telling us, the infiltration of psychiatry and allied professions into our work lives is not a progressive step in the health field, rather it signals the closer surveillance and social control of labour under neoliberal conditions. The following chapter moves on to discuss how the future workers have also become victims of this psychiatric hegemony through the closer monitoring of their behaviour in the education system.

Bibliography

Aho, K. (2010) 'The Psychopathology of American Shyness: A Hermeneutic Reading', *Journal for the Theory of Social Behaviour*, 40(2): 190–206.

American Psychiatric Association. (1980) *Diagnostic and Statistical Manual of Mental Disorders* (3rd ed.). Washington, DC: American Psychiatric Association.

American Psychiatric Association. (1987) *Diagnostic and Statistical Manual of Mental Disorders* (3rd ed. rev.). Washington, DC: American Psychiatric Association.

American Psychiatric Association. (2013) *Diagnostic and Statistical Manual of Mental Disorders* (5th ed.). Arlington, VA: American Psychiatric Association.

Brouillette, E. (2016) 'Why Therapists Should Talk Politics', *The New York Times*, http://mobile.nytimes.com/blogs/opinionator/2016/03/15/why-therapists-should-talk-politics/? (retrieved on 17 March 2016).

Brown, P. (1974) *Towards a Marxist Psychology*. New York: Harper & Row.

Cautin, R. L., Freedheim, D. K., and DeLeon, P. H. (2013) 'Psychology as a Profession', in Freedheim, D. K. (Ed.), *Handbook of Psychology, Volume 1: History of Psychology* (pp. 32–54). Hoboken, NJ: Wiley.

Conrad, P. (2007) *The Medicalization of Society: On the Transformation of Human Conditions into Treatable Disorders*. Baltimore: John Hopkins University Press.

Cottle, M. (1999) 'Selling Shyness: How Doctors and Drug Companies Created the "Social Phobia" Epidemic', *The New Republic*, http://www.antidepressantsfacts.com/selling-shyness.htm (retrieved on 20 April 2016).

Ehrenreich, B. (2009) *Smile or Die: How Positive Thinking Fooled America and the World*. London: Granta Publications.

Elraz, H. (2013) 'The "Sellable Semblance": Employability in the Context of Mental-Illness', *Ephemera: Theory & Politics in Organization*, 13(4): 809–824.

Farnham, A. (2014) '20 Fastest Growing Occupations', *ABC News*, http://abcnews.go.com/Business/americas-20-fastest-growing-jobs-surprise/story?id=22364716 (retrieved on 7 April 2016).

Foucault, M. (1988a) *Madness and Civilization: A History of Insanity in the Age of Reason*. New York: Vintage Books.

Gayle, D. (2015) 'Mental Health Workers Protest at Move to Integrate Clinic with Jobcentre', *The Guardian*, http://www.theguardian.com/society/2015/jun/26/mental-health-protest-clinic-jobcentre-streatham (retrieved on 11 April 2016).

Jonason, P. K., Jones, A., and Lyons, M. (2013) 'Creatures of the Night: Chronotypes and the Dark Triad Traits', *Personality and Individual Differences*, 55(5): 538–541.

Lane, C. (2007) *Shyness: How Normal Behavior Became a Sickness*. New Haven: Yale University Press.

Moynihan, R., and Cassels, A. (2005) *Selling Sickness: How Drug Companies are Turning Us All into Patients*. Crows Nest: Allen and Unwin.

Partnership for Workplace Mental Health. (2006) *A Mentally Healthy Workforce—It's Good for Business*. Arlington, VA: Partnership for Workplace Mental Health.

Roberts, R. (2015) *Psychology and Capitalism: The Manipulation of Mind*. Alresford: Zero Books.

Robinson, J. (1997) *The Failure of Psychiatry: A Marxist Critique*. London: Index Books.

Rose, N. (1999) *Governing the Soul: The Shaping of the Private Self* (2nd ed.). London: Free Association Books.

Rosenthal, S. (2010) *Sick and Sicker: Essays on Class, Health and Health Care*. Hamilton, ON: J.H. French & Company.

Rosenthal, S., and Campbell, P. (2016) *Marxism and Psychology*. Toronto: ReMarx Publishing.

Scott, S. (2004) 'The Shell, the Stranger and the Competent Other: Towards a Sociology of Shyness', *Sociology*, 38(1): 121–37.

Scott, S. (2006) 'The Medicalization of Shyness: From Social Misfits to Social Fitness', *Sociology of Health and Illness*, 28(2): 133–153.

Scull, A. (1989) *Social Order/Mental Disorder: Anglo-American Psychiatry in Historical Perspective*. Berkeley: University of California Press.

Scull, A. (1993) *The Most Solitary of Afflictions: Madness and Society in Britain, 1700–1900*. New Haven: Yale University Press.

Zimbardo, P. G. (1977) *Shyness: What It is, What To Do About It*. Reading, MA: Addison-Wesley.

5

Youth: Medicalising Deviance

This chapter considers the key economic and ideological factors within capitalist society that have precipitated what might be described as the relatively recent psychiatric and therapeutic "gold rush" of diagnosing young people with ever greater varieties of mental illness. As regimes of work have changed throughout the twentieth century and the demand for the workforce to possess higher and more complex skills has become greater, it will be shown that a focus on compulsory schooling justifies the closer surveillance and control of youth behaviour by psychiatric and associated professions. In forwarding the central argument of this book, a socio-historical analysis is performed on the diagnosis of ADHD, currently the most popular mental illness label given to school-aged children and young adults. While considering the issues of deinstitutionalisation, psy-professional struggles over jurisdiction, and the encroaching power of the pharmaceutical industry, the ADHD case study, along with textual analyses of consecutive DSMs, will show that the increasing infiltration of the psychiatric discourse into the education system serves a significant function for capitalism in enforcing dominant moral codes and economic prerogatives while pathologising any deviation or resistance to these patterns of authority.

B.M.Z. Cohen, *Psychiatric Hegemony*,
DOI 10.1057/978-1-137-46051-6_5

Wilkinson and Pickett (2010: 63) estimate that a million children in Britain are currently mentally ill, including one in ten of those aged between five and sixteen. Understanding these figures in the context of the education system, the scholars note that "in any secondary school with 1000 students, 50 will be severely depressed, 100 will be distressed, 10–20 will be suffering from obsessive-compulsive disorder and between 5–10 girls will have an eating disorder" (Wilkinson and Pickett 2010: 63). And the numbers appear to be growing. For example, in the case of attention-deficit/hyperactivity disorder (ADHD), three to five per cent of young people in the US were diagnosed with the disorder in 1970s (Conrad 2006: xi) whereas the current estimate is between seven and nine per cent of the youth population (Bowden 2014: 423). Recent studies from the US Centers for Disease Control and Prevention suggests an even higher rate of 11 per cent of school-age children, including 20 per cent of the male population (Saul 2014: 16). This represents a growth in ADHD in the US of 41 per cent in the last ten years (Saul 2014: 16). Whitaker and Cosgrove (2015: 92) estimate that 3.5 million young people in America are now being prescribed ADHD medication, which is "nearly six times the number in 1990."

As will be detailed later in this chapter, my analysis suggests that the range of mental disorders that can be associated with young people is currently 47 from a total of 374 classified in the DSM-5. Fifty years ago, in the first edition of the DSM, the figure was just eight. This impressive picture of the current "epidemic" of child mental illness can be contrasted with the knowledge that just a hundred years ago cases of mental disorder in children was considered most rare, with there being no specific pathology that psychiatry believed affected young people in particular (Timimi 2008: 166). How can we explain the increase in the rates and numbers of mental illnesses said to be afflicting young people across western society, especially over the past 35 years? Critical scholars have pointed to a number of factors including the consideration of psychiatrists as "moral entrepreneurs" responsible for the increased medicalisation of childhood, the need for a continual expansion of psy-professional activity into new areas of public and private life, and the role of pharmaceutical companies in distorting notions of "mental illness" to increase the profits from drug consumption (Rose 2006: 476–479). While the increasing medicalisation of deviant behaviour is a common theme within much of this scholarship, writers are cautious as to the seemingly complex dynamics whereby a specific aspect of young peoples' behaviour becomes categorised as a new mental illness by psychiatry (though pharmaceutical companies are often seen as a key agent here). Rose (2006: 480), however, has suggested that this medicalisation thesis should be tempered by a more "subtle" and less deterministic approach through which we can understand how both individuals and their doctors discursively code experience "in relation to a cultural norm of the active, responsible, choosing self, realizing his or her potential in the world through shaping a lifestyle."

The argument I develop here is much simpler than either Rose's or the medicalisation scholars, less subtle maybe, but certainly more straightforward: rates of mental illness for young people have increased because of capitalism's need to mould the moral character of the individual at an earlier age than previously. As the last chapter documented, neoliberalism has seen the progressive creep of psychiatry and associated professions into the workplace, training centres, and welfare and unemployment offices to enforce self-surveillance and progress "character building" in the interests of capitalism. Likewise, such regimes depoliticise and pathologise resistance through re-framing the systemic problems of an alienating and unfulfilling work environment as symptoms of "mental illness" and, thus, part of an individual's own failings. With the requirement for more compliant, competitive, and skilled citizens needed for the neoliberal marketplace, the psy-professionals have also intensified their focus on youth; this has particularly been achieved through the compulsory education system as the primary site for surveillance and, consequently, diagnostic expansion. This chapter begins by outlining the social construction of "children" and "young people," and the subsequent concern for their moral obligations by welfare agencies. It will then focus on the introduction of compulsory schooling as well as the development of child psychology and child psychiatric services which emerge from the education factories. Discussion of the post-war struggle for professional jurisdiction of disturbed and disabled children will be given, followed lastly by a detailed analysis of psychiatry's increasing focus on young people in neoliberal society.

The Social Construction of Childhood

At the end of the twentieth century, Rose (1999: 123) stated that childhood had become "the most intensively governed sector of personal existence." This includes the surveillance of the home and the school by health, welfare, and education services. It was not always this way; in fact, "childhood" as a separate and distinct phase of the life cycle only emerges with the Enlightenment and then develops further with industrial society (Aires 1962; Conrad and Schneider 1992: 145). Before this period, little attention was shown to these smaller versions of adults who were afforded the same rights and obligations as the rest of the population. Specifically, the nineteenth century saw key changes in this view, as birth and the first years of a person's life were reconceptualised as a period of significance to industrial citizens' future physical and moral health. The early years were reshaped as a time of "innocence" where the child needed special attention and guidance from authorities (Conrad and Schneider 1992: 146). Consequently, this period witnessed a growing concern for the younger population from the media, politicians, charities, and the public, which resulted in the emergence of professional groups and organisations specifically focused on childhood as a new "social issue." The construction and subsequent problematisation of young people in the nineteenth century can be succinctly understood as informed by two necessary conditions for the expansion of industrial capital at this time: firstly, the economic requirement for the labour force to be physically healthier, better skilled, better organised, and generally more conditioned to industrial work regimes prior to entering the factories and the mills. And secondly, the ideological requirement for the working classes to conform to the new industrial environment, embracing the dominant norms and values of capitalism without dissent (these ideas often being framed by religious groups, the media, and politicians as a concern for the "future morality" of society). As a result, there is an increase in the surveillance of the emerging nuclear family (Chap. 6). However, it is with the establishment of compulsory schooling in the latter decades of the nineteenth century that these economic and ideological prerogatives are given their clearest and most enduring form.

The establishment of compulsory education addressed the need for a more literate and higher skilled workforce (Timimi 2008: 165), while at the same time allaying the fears of the ruling classes as to the perceived threat of an increasingly organised and politicised working class population. The new public schools system therefore performed a secondary socialisation function, instilling dominant codes in the future labour force and acting as a site where authority and moral obligation of the new citizens could be enforced. Similar to the factory, the asylum, and the prison, the school established another institution of social control in industrial society where obedience to the social order could be reinforced, primarily through surveillance by moral authorities rather than through physical punishment. Citing John Locke's philosophy on education which informed this state apparatus, Scull (1993: 108) notes that "[t]he child needed to be taught to be 'his own slave driver'" through rewarding "appropriate" behaviour and shaming deviant actions. Joined by an emergent teaching profession, the psychological sciences would come to take a decisive role in enforcing this ideological function of the education system.

Following the enactment of legislation in the 1830s to outlaw child labour in Britain (Duffin 2000: 330), the increased visibility on the streets along with public concern as to the potential delinquency of the young working class population led to demands that greater attention be paid to child welfare. Informed by Christian and nationalist doctrines as well as burgeoning psychological, educational, and philosophical approaches to "child development" (Timimi 2008: 165), many "child-saving" charities and philanthropic groups emerged during this period to campaign for greater social and medical interventions in early life, with a particular focus on the family and the school. As Conrad and Schneider (1992: 146) recount, "[t]hese reformers, including moralists, educators, and clergy, supported child-rearing philosophies that emphasized psychological control and moral solicitude, in the name of benefiting the child." For such reformers, a great deal of momentum was gained from the introduction of compulsory schooling—this led to what Timimi (2008: 165) calls "a prolonged and unprecedented public discussion about the physical and mental condition of children." This concern for the psychological well-being and development of the young citizen also paralleled the more general growth of public medicine in Victorian Britain. As Porter (1997: 633–634) has outlined of the guiding principles,

> medicine (it was argued) had to become a positive and systematic enterprise, undertaking planned surveillance of apparently healthy, normal people as well as the sick, tracing groups from infancy to old age, logging the incidence of chronic, inherited and constitutional conditions, correlating ill health against variables like income, education, class, diet and housing.

By the end of the nineteenth century, the medical gaze had expanded to incorporate "the entire psycho-social economy" of society (Porter 1997: 634), including a growing interest in education. Within the school environment, the concern for the "morality" of the future workers shown earlier by child-saving groups became a focus for the scientific surveillance and management of young people by the psychological sciences under the auspices of identifying learning difficulties and behavioural problems. In the new century, psychiatrists and psychologists began to observe, monitor, and evaluate the classroom, not for mental pathologies within the child but for behaviour that differentiated them from the "normal" and the expected. Thus the psy-professionals' interventions in schools were, from the beginning, moral rather than scientific judgements of appropriate behaviour, holding within them the aim of enforcing dominant and desired notions of "normality" on the young. As Rose (1999: 133) has summarised,

> It is around pathological children—the troublesome, the recalcitrant, the delinquent—that conceptions of normality have taken shape. It is not that a knowledge of the normal course of development of the child has enabled experts to become more skilled at identifying those unfortunate children who are in some way abnormal. Rather, expert notions of normality are extrapolated from our attention to those children who worry the courts, teachers, doctors, and parents. Normality is not an observation but a valuation. It contains not only a judgment about what is desirable, but an injunction as to the goal to be achieved. In so doing, the very notion of "the normal" today awards power to scientific truth and expert authority.

Before the advent of compulsory schooling it had been rare for children to be conceptualised as suffering from a "mental illness," though Timimi (2008: 166) notes that there were occasional youth admittances to asylums throughout the nineteenth century. However, the concern for the welfare of the child and the general "mental hygiene" of the population in the early part of the twentieth century changed this view and saw the emergence of medical and social disciplines and professional bodies that, for the first time, specialised in child and adolescent health, including the establishment of paediatrics as a sub-discipline of medicine (Duffin 2000: 317). Similarly, early development psychology and child psychiatry were also established (Timimi 2008: 166), the latter notably helped by the foundation in England of the Tavistock Square Clinic in 1920 which boasted a children's department responsible for promoting "awareness" of childhood mental disorders (Porter 1997: 645).

"Intelligence" Testing

In the previous chapter I discussed the development of an increasingly complex work environment throughout the twentieth century; at the same time, the psychological sciences expanded its areas of jurisdiction to facilitate skills diversification and "personal development," increase the productivity and efficiency of the workforce, and enforce conformity to the dominant values of capital by pathologising and depoliticising worker resistance. The primary site for enforcing such structures of discipline on the future workforce, however, would come to be the school—this was where the psychological sciences would first make a significant claim to expertise beyond the psychiatric institution and the analyst's couch. Rose (1999: 135) recounts that, as with the factory or the parade ground, school brought children together in a single space where they could be observed and judged *en masse*. Individual differences between children were made visible by the school system, and the institution, "sought to discipline [children] according to institutional criteria and objectives" (Rose 1999: 140). However, there were those who would not or could not adapt to the desired moral codes for behaviour and performance at school. These young people—who came to be labelled as "educational imbeciles or the feeble-minded" (Rose 1999: 140)—were a problem for the authorities.

Inspired by the eugenicists' obsession for marking and testing biological and mental differences within the general population (Chap. 7), psychologists developed the intelligence quotient (IQ) test to measure the academic performance of school children and separate the able from the less-abled students. This is the beginning of psychometric and associated testing which has since expanded across many areas of economic and social life. Commenting on the significance of the "intelligence" test, Rose (1999: 143) states that,

> The technique of the test was the most important contribution of the psychological sciences to the human technologies of the first half of the twentieth century. The test routinizes the complex ensemble of social judgement on individual variability into an automatic device that makes difference visible and notable.

Thus, the intelligence test can be seen as a moral technology used specifically for the social judgement of school children by psychologists under the guise of "science" (see also Roberts 2015: 12–13). The inventor of the test, Alfred Binet, had developed it to identify the "feeble-minded" to be sent to special schools. Significant for contextualising later mass testings and screenings of school children for intelligence, abnormalities, and mental disorders, Rose (1999: 142, emphasis added) notes, "Binet's test used criteria that were directly educational and behavioural. *They were direct assessments of the degree of adaptation of individual children to the expectation that others had of them.*" The key to the success of Binet's test was not the ability to accurately measure "intelligence"—which he felt was impossible to predict through such time-restricted tests—but its administrative usefulness in identifying problematic individuals (Rose 1999: 142). By the 1960s, the "science" of testing school children had expanded to such an extent that it was enshrined in the United States under the federal Medicare package, where children could be screened for a whole host of physical and behavioural disorders. With mass-screening programmes administered through schools, Conrad and Schneider (1992: 155) state that it had become, "possible to establish diagnosis and intervention with deviant children to an extent beyond the dreams of the 19th-century child-savers." Under the pretext of "health care" for school children, these moral technologies aided the expansion of the psy-professionals into the education system over the course of the twentieth century, and with it an increased focus on childhood deviance and the use of psychiatric labels to neutralise such threats to authority.

The Rise of the Risky Kid

An analysis of successive editions of the DSM for youth-related diagnoses demonstrates three key issues to support my argument for the development of psychiatric hegemony here. Firstly, psychiatry has linked childhood mental illness to unwanted behaviour and conduct in the classroom from the very first edition. For example, the DSM-I introduced "learning disturbance" as a category of "special symptoms/reaction" (American Psychiatric Association 1952: 39), as well as the mental disorder of conduct disorder/disturbance (American Psychiatric Association 1952: 41) which included the example of truancy as symptomatic behaviour (in an updated form, the latter remains in the DSM-5) (see Appendix B for the full diagnostic list identified in each DSM). Secondly, the pathologisation of youth behaviour and the experiences/events of childhood and adolescence have increased exponentially, from eight diagnostic categories in the DSM-I to 47 in the DSM-5 (see Table 5.1). Young people have been a market of serious growth for the mental health industry, and psychiatry (along with pharmaceutical companies and other vested parties) has been successful in grabbing a significant piece of that pie over the years. From my analysis of the DSMs, the classifications and discourse on youth have grown considerably, divorcing all other areas of specific

Table 5.1 Number of youth-related diagnostic categories in the DSM, 1952–2013[a]

DSM-I (1952)	DSM-II (1968)	DSM-III (1980)	DSM-III-R (1987)	DSM-IV (1994)	DSM-IV-TR (2000)	DSM-5 (2013)
8	18	37	41	42	43	47

[a]See Appendix B for full diagnostic list.

psychiatric expansion. Thirdly, the growth in youth-related mental illness classifications and discourse is uneven, with the most pronounced increase evidenced in 1980 with the publication of the DSM-III. At the end of institutionalisation and the beginning of neoliberalism, the number of mental disorders aimed at young people and adolescents doubled from 18 in the DSM-II to 37 in the DSM-III. It is here, for example, that the behaviours of stuttering and being mute become mental illnesses (the former remains in the DSM-5 as childhood-onset fluency disorder (American Psychiatric Association 2013: 45–47)), while learning disabilities, social ineptitude, and (especially) boys' unruly behaviour are medicalised under labels such as autism and ADHD. In previous DSMs, references to "school" were rare (the word was mentioned only four times in the diagnostic categories in the DSM-I and twice in the DSM-II), yet in the DSM-III the word was liberally scattered across many diagnoses as both examples and the focus for a site of disorder, with the phrase being used a total of 91 times. Many new words and phrases associated with youth, education, and leisure were introduced under classifications and symptomologies in the DSM-III, and these have usually increased with each successive edition of the manual (see Table 5.2).

To fully understand the growth in the psychiatric surveillance of young people during the post-war period, it is necessary to consider the expansion of the welfare state in western societies, the struggle for control of

Table 5.2 Number of youth-related words/phrases in the DSM, 1952–2013[a]

Word/phrase	DSM-I (1952)	DSM-II (1968)	DSM-III (1980)	DSM-III-R (1987)	DSM-IV (1994)	DSM-IV-TR (2000)	DSM-5 (2013)
Adolescent/ce	9	39	211	274	206	216	179
Child/ren/hood	32	71	672	762	822	855	1318
Educat/ed/ion	0	0	6	4	14	16	26
Game/s/ing	0	0	6	12	12	12	75
Play/ing/mates	0	0	27	37	66	59	87
School	4	2	91	105	158	170	257
Teach/er/es/ing	0	0	8	6	12	19	18
Youth/young people	0	0	3	6	4	6	23
Total count	45	112	1024	1206	1294	1353	1983

[a]See Appendix A for methodology.

expertise over the areas of youth mental health and "mental retardation" between psychologists, psychiatrists, psychoanalysts, educationalists and social workers, societal concerns over the morality of young people, and the perceived increases in teenage delinquency and crime at the time. The expansion of intelligence testing to increasingly younger populations allowed for the detection of ever greater numbers of those considered "feeble-minded" or "morons." Confined to institutions for the "mentally retarded" or in "special schools," Eyal et al. (2010: 78–79) note that these "socially incapable" individuals were inevitably from working class and minority backgrounds, with professional judgements made on the basis of prevailing ideas of "feeble-mindedness" as related to delinquency and crime. The number of young people admitted to institutions for the mentally deficient increased dramatically between the 1940s and the 1960s, with Eyal et al. (2010: 114) recording a figure for America of 108,500 pupils in 1948 but 540,000 students by 1966 (the general school-age population in the country less than doubled over the same period). This period of intense institutionalisation of large numbers of young people represents the attempt of psy-professionals to exert social control over deviant groups who could be diverted from the public schools system into spaces of moral management and confinement. Being "mentally deficient" was a useful metaphor for deviant and troublesome individuals in the education system, as Eyal et al. (2010: 79) remarks, "[t]ruancy, delinquency, epilepsy, alcoholism, sexual promiscuity, even masturbation, all served as pretexts for commitment as mentally deficient, and the category of 'defective delinquent' was the main prism through which the problem of feeble-mindedness was viewed." Such moral failings of the post-war juvenile delinquent were conceptualised by child psychiatrists as evidence of a serious mental disorder (most often utilising the label of "childhood schizophrenia") for which they typically recommended psychiatric institutionalisation and a course of 20 ECT treatments (Eyal et al. 2010: 134).

As has been previously discussed in Chap. 3, deinstitutionalisation led to a significant change in the diagnostic focus of psychiatry from "severe and acute" mental illnesses—which typically called for an institutional response—to less severe pathologies which expanded their areas of expertise and locus of operations. By the mid-1970s there was a similar decline in the use of institutions for the "mentally retarded"—children were "mainstreamed" back into the public schools system and, consequently, a greater surveillance of young people within the education system by psychiatry and related professions unfolded. By the time of the publication of the DSM-III in 1980, youth-related mental illnesses had mysteriously doubled and delinquent behaviour such as pyromania, kleptomania, and other "conduct disorders" had been given their own DSM classifications. Thus, the DSM-III and the growing focus on youth mental illness can be understood as a consequence of the deinstitutionalisation of deviant youth from special education facilities. As with the move towards "milder" mental disorders in the community, the integration of children and young people once labelled as suffering from "learning disturbances" into mainstream schools called for the greater surveillance and control of youth behaviour in the wider education system. The increase in the psychiatric labelling of groups of young people with diagnoses such as oppositional defiant disorder, ADHD, conduct disorder, and autism is a consequence of the change in the site of psy-professional operations which, in the latter case, is supported by Eyal et al. (2010) who argue that the recent autism "epidemic" in western society is a result of the diagnostic substitution of the term "mentally retarded" for the more recent psychiatric label.

Education Factories and the Surveillance of the Future Workforce

In the mid-1970s my own primary school introduced a rule banning a popular lunchtime activity of inserting baked beans into bread rolls. We were instructed to eat rolls with butter only; the baked beans had to remain on the plate, outside the roll at all times. One day, a friend of mine disobeyed this rule and was caught by a teacher at our lunch table. The teacher was most put out by this open display of beans-in-roll pleasure. I was ten years old but even then curious about how the world worked, so I asked the teacher why this activity was forbidden. This was a mistake. The response was very loud and a bit scary. The lesson we learned that day was if there is something worse than blatantly disobeying school rules it was questioning them; students who question orders are by extension questioning authority. As outlined earlier in this chapter, compulsory education serves both an economic and an ideological function in capitalist society. Students learn a range of literacy and numeracy skills which will benefit the market in due course and, at the same time, they learn to conform, obey, and take for granted the norms and values of capitalist society as inscribed through the formal and informal processes of schooling. As neoliberalism has impacted compulsory schooling over the past 35 years, the latter ideological function has become increasingly important, with noted scholar and school teacher John Taylor Gatto (2002: 21) bluntly stating that "[n]o one believes that scientists are trained in science classes or politicians in civics classes or poets in English classes. The truth is that schools don't really teach anything except how to obey orders."

Schools manage the ideological reproduction of the future labour force. Youth dissent and resistance must be neutralised in the interests of enforcing the ideals of the ruling classes upon all young citizens. Rather than an array of free-thinking individuals, schools use techniques of scientific management on young people to produce "formulaic human beings whose behavior can be predicted and controlled" (Gatto 2002: 23). Difference or digressions from the expected behaviour are signs of deviance and can be consequently labelled as "learning difficulties" and signs of pathology. In western society, explains Adams (2008: 114), the education system rewards cohesion and cooperation with teachers, school rules, and the prescribed tasks of the classroom. Yet—as with the rules of my own primary school—the judging of the behaviour of pupils and how far they are "cooperating" or otherwise with teachers' expectations are context specific rather than universal. Instead of considering reactions to behaviour considered as inappropriate and incorrect as a product of the professional expectations of teachers alone, Adams (2008: 114) argues we need to place them in their broader socio-political and cultural context. The current ideal type among teachers for the conforming and non-confrontational pupil needs to be seen as a result and reinforcement of this wider context. Thus, "inappropriate" behaviour does not necessarily reflect impairment but rather "socio-cultural and political actions" of the wider policy environment. "Dominant political positions," states Adams (2008: 114), "contribute to the creation of categories such as 'deviant' through their description of appropriate and inappropriate. This duly positions professional response that in turn can and does further legitimate policy."

The psychological sciences have become increasingly useful for teachers and the schools system in supporting the exclusion of troublesome pupils and labelling non-conformist students as mentally disturbed. Szasz has previously highlighted the absurd vagueness of diagnostic symptomology which allows any aspect of child behaviour in the classroom to be understood as a potential mental disorder. This he does by citing a journal article from 1962 which argued for more psychiatric services in the education system, identifying the following symptoms which suggested underlying pathologies in school children:

> 1. Academic problems—under-achievement, over-achievement, erratic, uneven performance. 2. Social problems with siblings, peers—such as the aggressive child, the submissive child, the show-off. 3. Relations with parental and other authority figures, such as defiant behavior, submissive behavior, ingratiation. 4. Overt behavioral manifestations, such as tics, nail-biting, thumb-sucking ... [and] interests more befitting to the opposite sex (such as tom-boy girl and effeminate boy). (Radin, cited in Szasz 1997: 35).

As signalled by the recent construction of mental illness categories explicitly focused on student behaviour in school (such as losing homework and failing to pay attention in class), psy-professionals' role in the public education system has become more pronounced over the past few decades. Just as profound, however, has been the heightened concentration in the post-welfare era on the school as a site of economic competition, with market forces more directly influencing school management, teaching processes, and ultimately the pressures placed on young people to acquire greater numbers of qualifications and skills than previously. Adams (2008: 115) has described how neoliberal education policies have subordinated the needs of individual students to the wider economy, arguing that "in effect, 'learner' became 'worker in waiting' with the knowledge and skills deemed as worthwhile to gleam from school as those required and celebrated in the commercial world." As a result, commentators have noted how schools have become far more demanding social environments which involve greater levels of self-regulation of young people (Timimi 2009: 139). As western governments have demanded greater numbers of students continue in education and re-orientate themselves to a future as white-collar workers, the qualities of school pupils once considered appropriate (such as exuberance, curiosity, and energy) have been replaced by more on-task academic learning and seat-work (Graham 2008: 24). As a result of the pressures on teachers and pupils in this neoliberal environment, there has been a need for a closer surveillance of behaviour in school and, more readily, a desire to discipline the defiant child through the application of various mental illness labels. As the Department for Education and Skills for England and Wales stated in 2005, "better discipline … [in schools will] enable teachers to teach and learners to learn" (cited in Adams 2008: 115). To further illustrate how psychiatric hegemony has been achieved as a result of the needs of capital to ideologically control young citizens, the following section profiles the origins and development of ADHD, the most popular label of mental disorder currently applied to young people.

Case Study: Attention-Deficit/Hyperactivity Disorder

As noted at the beginning of the chapter, up to 11 per cent of school-age children in the United States are currently diagnosed with ADHD (Saul 2014: 16). Granted, these figures are considerably higher than those for other western countries. For example, Zwi et al. (in Conrad 2006: xii) suggest that the United States has a diagnosis rate for ADHD some 10–30 times higher than that for the UK. However, one trend which unites all western societies is the increased use of the label for problematic children over time—particularly since the 1990s (Conrad 2006: xii)—and the increased use of stimulant medications as a treatment option. The dominant biomedical view states that ADHD is a neurological dysfunction of the brain. This is despite a lack of any evidence for the biological causation of the disorder (Christian 1997: 34; DeGrandpre 2000: 9). A brief overview of the symptoms for the mental disorder in the DSM-5 highlights the obvious psychiatric construction of ADHD as a set of education markers—to which has been added workplace markers (Chap. 4)—of deviance and failure within the schooling system. The symptomologies given by the American Psychiatric Association (2013: 59) for the "inattention" markers of ADHD are,

> a. Often fails to give close attention to details or makes careless mistakes in schoolwork, at work, or during other activities (e.g., overlooks or misses details, work is inaccurate).
>
> b. Often has difficulty sustaining attention in tasks or play activities (e.g., has difficulty remaining focused during lectures, conversations, or lengthy reading).
>
> c. Often does not seem to listen when spoken to directly (e.g., mind seems elsewhere, even in the absence of any obvious distraction).
>
> d. Often does not follow through on instructions and fails to finish schoolwork, chores, or duties in the workplace (e.g., starts tasks but quickly loses focus and is easily sidetracked).
>
> e. Often has difficulty organizing tasks and activities (e.g., difficulty managing sequential tasks; difficulty keeping materials and belongings in order; messy, disorganized work; has poor time management; fails to meet deadlines).
>
> f. Often avoids, dislikes, or is reluctant to engage in tasks that require sustained mental effort (e.g., schoolwork or homework; for older adolescents and adults, preparing reports, completing forms, reviewing lengthy papers).
>
> g. Often loses things necessary for tasks or activities (e.g., school materials, pencils, books, tools, wallets, keys, paperwork, eyeglasses, mobile telephones).
>
> h. Is often easily distracted by extraneous stimuli (for older adolescents and adults, may include unrelated thoughts).
>
> i. Is often forgetful in daily activities (e.g., doing chores, running errands; for older adolescents and adults, returning calls, paying bills, keeping appointments).

As a general marker of productivity, changes to the ADHD diagnosis between DSM-IV (1994) and DSM-5 (2013) have focused on expanding the diagnosis to adults by introducing aspects of work and home life as additional realms for symptomologies. Similarly, the symptoms from the American Psychiatric Association (2013: 60) for the "hyperactivity and impulsivity" component of ADHD are,

a. Often fidgets with or taps hands or feet or squirms in seat.

b. Often leaves seat in situations when remaining seated is expected (e.g., leaves his or her place in the classroom, in the office or other workplace, or in other situations that require remaining in place).

c. Often runs about or climbs in situations where it is inappropriate. (Note: In adolescents or adults, may be limited to feeling restless.)

d. Often unable to play or engage in leisure activities quietly.

e. Is often "on the go," acting as if "driven by a motor" (e.g., is unable to be or uncomfortable being still for extended time, as in restaurants, meetings; may be experienced by others as being restless or difficult to keep up with).

f. Often talks excessively.

g. Often blurts out an answer before a question has been completed (e.g., completes people's sentences; cannot wait for turn in conversation).

h. Often has difficulty waiting his or her turn (e.g., while waiting in line).

i. Often interrupts or intrudes on others (e.g., butts into conversations, games, or activities; may start using other people's things without asking or receiving permission; for adolescents and adults, may intrude into or take over what others are doing).

Clear within the phraseology and the "symptoms" of ADHD is the concern to medicalise the behaviour of unruly children in the classroom; it is a question of children refusing to conform to the required order of school life and, therefore, the APA developing the label of ADHD as a device of social control (rather than a product of scientific enquiry). As Graham (2008: 23) has correctly remarked of these symptomologies, "most of the behaviours listed are connected to (and one could even argue contingent upon) the demands of schooling." The contradiction between the espousal of biological aetiology and treatment of increasing numbers of young people, and the obvious place of compulsory education in the construction of the ADHD label has been further highlighted by Christian (1997: 34) when he states that "[s]chool classrooms have had and still have an intimate connection to the origination and the diagnosis of ADHD; and yet, little attention is given to the school setting in the causal explanation of the disorder." Rafalovich (2004: 21–34) has sought to partially address this situation by performing a socio-historical analysis of pre-ADHD labels, in the process detailing psychiatry's increased focus on the "morality" of young people's behaviour in school at the end of the nineteenth century.

The growing medical concern for the "moral imbecile" was specifically contemplated by the physician George Still at the beginning of the twentieth century when he gave a series of lectures at the Royal College of Physicians in London, arguing for the increased scientific investigation of "the occurrence of defective moral control as a morbid condition in children" (cited in Rafalovich 2004: 27). Still believed morality to have a biological base, so pathology could be suspected if it appeared that children were not developing in the way society had designated (i.e., if it appeared that the appropriate moral controls on the child's behaviour were absent). However, he argued that such children should not to be confused with the "retarded" or "idiot" child. Following his own observations, he stated that these young people were just as intelligent as those who showed moral control and thus demonstrated a degree of agency in their immorality. Symptoms of these defective young people included "passionateness," "lawlessness," and "wanton mischievousness-destructiveness" (cited in Rafalovich 2004: 28). Too young for prison and too smart to be considered an imbecile, Still argued that this was a hereto under-investigated and under-theorised group of juvenile delinquents who offered a potential threat to the future of society. Despite the clear linkage between medical science and dominant views on morality within Still's work, official historians of psychiatry continue to see the physician as a scientific visionary, responsible for the original research on children which would eventually lead to the modern classification of ADHD. In contrast, Rafalovich (2004) identifies the growing concern for deviant and unruly youth by the medical profession as the origins of the current DSM label.

Significant to Rafalovich's (2004: 29–34) socio-historical analysis is the diagnosis of encephalitis lethargica (EL)—commonly known as "sleepy sickness"—which concerned medicine in the 1920s. Admittedly a poorly defined illness, EL can be understood as an early explanation for delinquency, including as it did the symptoms of "emotional instability, irritability, ... lying, thieving, impaired memory and attention, personal untidiness, tics, ... poor motor control, and general hyperactivity" (Kessler, cited in Rafalovich 2004: 30). Similar to Still, the physician

Roger Kennedy utilised case studies to argue that the young people suffering from EL were in fact, "moral rather than mental imbeciles. Some of them appear dull and drowsy, but in their antics and behaviour they display a cunning that is not commensurate with greatly impaired mental faculties" (cited in Rafalovich 2004: 32). As Rafalovich (2004: 30) argues, such statements exemplify a crucial point in the construction of the ADHD diagnosis, where child psychiatry begins to use specific diagnoses such as EL to claim that "persistently defiant childhood behaviour represented physiological pathology."

Such claims as to the biological aetiology of the child's immoral character appeared to be confirmed during the 1930s when the synthesising and marketing of new psychoactive drugs saw an expansion—especially in the United States—in the scope and influence of pharmaceutical industries on the psychological sciences and the general public (Conrad 1975: 14). In 1937, Charles Bradley presented the results of a drugs study on school children with learning disabilities. His research appeared to show that amphetamines, paradoxically, calmed many of his participants and allowed them to complete study tasks with less disruption. Now an often-cited study in the development of drug treatments for ADHD, at the time it was treated as no more than a curiosity. Bradley's study was performed on children already attending special institutions and diagnosed with "learning disabilities," thus the results of the research appeared from the outside as if it was only relevant to a small cohort of young people who had already been excluded from mainstream schooling. Yet, an interest in improving student "discipline" in schools by the psychological sciences and pharmaceutical researchers—under the guise of helping those with "learning difficulties"—slowly progressed over the following decades. In the 1950s, the first edition of DSM named a number of mental disorders which directly referred to young people's deviant behaviour at school (such as conduct disturbance, see American Psychiatric Association 1952: 41) and the drug Ritalin appeared on the US market for the first time. Following the development of Laufer et al.'s new diagnostic category of hyperkinetic impulse disorder in 1957 (Conrad 1975: 14), the turbulence of the 1960s led to an increase in disruptive and resistant young people being labelled as hyperactive. In 1968, the APA more than doubled their diagnostic categories for young people with the publication of the DSM-II, including a dedicated section on "behavior disorders of childhood and adolescence" (American Psychiatric Association 1968: 49–51). Among the new disorders was hyperkinetic reaction of childhood (or adolescence), which the APA described as characterised by "overactivity, restlessness, distractibility, and short attention span" (American Psychiatric Association 1968: 50). With the help of "moral entrepreneurs" such as pharmaceutical companies and the Association for Children with Learning Disabilities (Conrad 1975: 16), by the mid-1970s hyperkinesis had become "the most common child psychiatric problem" in the United States (Conrad 1975: 14).

As has been noted earlier in this chapter, a significant shift occurred with the production of the DSM-III in 1980. While deinstitutionalisation was a threat to public psychiatry, the relatively small field of child psychiatry offered opportunities for the expansion of the medical discipline into new areas of work and expertise. With the mainstreaming of deviant children who were once confined to "special schools" and the increasing requirement for adolescents to upskill and study beyond the end of compulsory schooling, the interests of the state in managing and controlling youth within the education system coincides with the specific interests of the psy-professionals to expand their areas of influence beyond one institution and into another.

Reflecting on the DSM-III committee's desire to open up the possibility of mental disorders to a much broader population—some might say everyone—a whole chapter of the manual is devoted to "disorders usually *first evident* in infancy, childhood, or adolescence" (American Psychiatric Association 1980: 35, emphasis added). Taking up five pages of this chapter was the new diagnosis of attention deficit disorder (ADD) which, under the two subtypes of ADD with hyperactivity and ADD without hyperactivity, brought together numerous previous labels given to troublesome children (including hyperkinesis and minimal brain dysfunction). Significant here was the growing emphasis placed upon the *inattentiveness* of the school child (examples in the DSM-III included that the child, "often fails to finish things," "often doesn't seem to listen," is "easily distracted," and "has difficulty concentrating on schoolwork" (American Psychiatric Association 1980: 43)), a focus that should not only be seen in the cynical context of diagnostic expansion—a move from explicitly disruptive behaviour to simple levels of concentration at school—but also in terms of the changing needs of the classroom towards more studious and attentive pupils. Reflecting this change, ADD became the now familiar classification of ADHD in the revised edition of the DSM-III seven years later (American Psychiatric Association 1987: 50–53). Following his extensive research on ADHD with clinicians, parents, teachers, and pupils, Rafalovich (2004: 131) finds that key to "discovering" behaviour that will consequently be defined by authorities as ADHD is the child's school. Such behaviour, he states, is "articulated in one of two ways: as academic struggles, denoting an inability to competently engage in the achievement of classroom assignments, and as social struggles, denoting interpersonal conflicts with other students and/or teachers" (Rafalovich 2004: 131). These two sites of struggle at school are then reflected in the symptomology constructed by psychiatry within the ADHD diagnosis, as Rafalovich (2004: 131) concludes, "the disorder's inattention component can be seen in academic failure, and its hyperactivity component can be witnessed in children's overt behavioral problems."

With the construction and expansion of the ADHD category to greater numbers of young people, the emphasis is changing from overt disruption to student inattention. This can be seen as reflecting the changing educational priorities in neoliberalism from the social control of deviant working class youth to the ideological enforcement of a dominant morality on the broader population of school children. The move towards consideration of simple inattention as pathology has also had the interesting by-product of slowly closing the gender gap of this still male-dominated mental disorder (DeGrandpre 2000: 147). Following prescribed gender behaviour, boys have been more likely to be labelled as loud, aggressive troublemakers in class, while girls have been considered by teachers as more passive and introspective. Thus, Rafalovich (2004: 125, emphasis added) rightly summates that "[t]he issue at the core of why there is such a huge gender discrepancy in instances of ADHD has more to do with *behavioral visibility* than with the actual existence of the condition." The diagnosing of boys with ADHD has been estimated as three to five times higher than for girls (DeGrandpre 2000: 147), a situation that led the *New York Times* in 1994 to conclude that boyhood was in danger of becoming a "state of proto-disease" (cited in DeGrandpre 2000: 147).

Increasing the focus on inattention in subsequent editions of the DSM has been a useful way in which the APA can attempt to address the above gender bias in the application of the ADHD label. In his book *Saving Normal*, the chair of the DSM-IV task force, Allen Frances (2013: 142), freely admits of the classification that "[w]e changed a few words so that the definition [of ADHD] would be more female friendly—taking into account that girls are more likely to be inattentive 'space cadets' and less likely than boys to be hyperactive." Apart from glimpsing another picture of the impressive manner in which the DSM task forces undertake their work (i.e., a reliance on dominant, common sense notions of "appropriate" gender roles rather than any scientific evidence), Frances' statement highlights the blatant intention of the APA to expand the classification outwards to groups currently under-represented in the profile of ADHD.

In conclusion, this socio-historical analysis of ADHD has demonstrated that the diagnosis emerged from the closer focus of the psy-professions on the morality of young people in the twentieth century and the concern for controlling and correcting deviant behaviour. The expansion of ADHD from a rare disorder to a popular disease among young people over the past 35 years can be understood as a result of capitalism's need to enforce discipline, compliance, and authority on the future workforce at a younger age. The redefined standards of normality in the neoliberal classroom are therefore designated under the lexicon of psychiatric hegemony as a concern for the control, correction, and treatment of deviant groups of children. ADHD as a classic example of the medicalisation of deviant behaviour is perhaps best summed up by a special education teacher cited in Rafalovich's (2004: 111) research who, without irony, states that "[t]he last thing someone with untreated ADHD wants to do is go to school."

Summary

Rose (1999: 123) has commented on the importance of young people to industrial society that "the child—as an idea and a target—has become inextricably connected to the aspirations of authorities." Over time, psychiatric authorities have medicalised more and more aspects of the experiences and behaviour of children. From intelligence testing and the institutionalisation of "mentally deficient" children to DSM-III and the demands of the current education system, this chapter has explored the expansion of psy-professionals' focus on children and adolescents over the past hundred years. Through socio-historical investigation, analysis of consecutive DSMs as well as utilising the case study of ADHD, I have demonstrated how the supposed "experts on the mind" have served to reinforce the economic and ideological prerogatives of the capitalist class. For youth, this primarily takes place through compulsory schooling as secondary socialisers of the future workforce. Throughout the development of industrial capitalism it has been demonstrated that the psy-professionals has been concerned with the perceived immorality of working class youth. The psychiatric discourse previously pathologised such deviant behaviour through incarcerating such groups in "special schools" and then, more recently, through the construction of an increasing range of mental disorders aimed specifically at youth and schooling. As Rafalovich (2004: 64) has concluded, from the diagnosis of EL nearly a hundred years ago to ADHD currently, the institutional location has been a key variable in understanding the construction of childhood mental illness. He states that "problems in school have been historically seen as indicative of severe social maladjustment, and improvement in school performance is equated to 'appropriate' social behaviour" (Rafalovich 2004: 64). As framed by the neoliberal focus on the individual as the site of change, the institutional requirements of the school for conformity and compliance means that now more than ever teachers are aided by the mental health system. The focus of teachers on the notion of the "individual deficit" of young people, comments Adams (2008: 123), should now be seen as having "become even more political rather than psychological."

Speaking more generally to the drivers of the medicalisation of deviant behaviour in his classic study of hyperactive children, Conrad (2006: 98) states that "[t]he greater the benefit to established institutions, the greater the likelihood of medicalization." While the changing demands of capitalism brought about the relatively recent expansion in psy-professional activity focused on young people, the discussion in the next chapter investigates an institution of industrial society which has experienced psy-professional intervention for a more sustained length of time, namely the family. It will be demonstrated that the reconstituted nuclear family system in capitalist society has served to confine and oppress women for specific economic reasons, and that this system of patriarchal relations has been constantly reinforced by psy-professional practice over time.

Bibliography

Adams, P. (2008) 'Positioning Behaviour: Attention Deficit/Hyperactivity Disorder (ADHD) in the Post-Welfare Educational Era', *International Journal of Inclusive Education*, 12(2): 113–125.

Aires, P. (1962) *Centuries of Childhood*. New York: Vintage Books.

American Psychiatric Association. (1952) *Diagnostic and Statistical Manual: Mental Disorders*. Washington, DC: American Psychiatric Association.

American Psychiatric Association. (1968) *Diagnostic and Statistical Manual of Mental Disorders* (2nd ed.). Washington, DC: American Psychiatric Association.

American Psychiatric Association. (1980) *Diagnostic and Statistical Manual of Mental Disorders* (3rd ed.). Washington, DC: American Psychiatric Association.

American Psychiatric Association. (1987) *Diagnostic and Statistical Manual of Mental Disorders* (3rd ed. rev.). Washington, DC: American Psychiatric Association.

American Psychiatric Association. (2013) *Diagnostic and Statistical Manual of Mental Disorders* (5th ed.). Arlington, VA: American Psychiatric Association.

Bowden, G. (2014) 'The Merit of Sociological Accounts of Disorder: The Attention-Deficit Hyperactivity Disorder Case', *Health*, 18(4): 422–438.

Christian, J. M. (1997) 'The Body as a Site of Reproduction and Resistance: Attention Deficit Hyperactivity Disorder and the Classroom', *Interchange*, 28(1): 31–43.

Conrad, P. (1975) 'The Discovery of Hyperkinesis: Notes on the Medicalization of Deviant Behaviour', *Social Problems*, 23(1): 12–21.

Conrad, P. (2006) *Identifying Hyperactive Children: The Medicalization of Deviant Behavior* (rev. ed.). Aldershot: Ashgate.

Conrad, P., and Schneider, J. (1992) *Deviance and Medicalization: From Badness to Sickness*. Philadelphia: Temple University Press.

DeGrandpre, R. J. (2000) *Ritalin Nation: Rapid-Fire Culture and the Transformation of Human Consciousness* (rev. ed.). New York: W.W. Norton & Company.

Duffin, J. (2000) *History of Medicine: A Scandalously Short Introduction.* Houndmills, Basingstoke: Macmillan.

Eyal, G., Hart, B., Onculer, E., Oren, N., and Rossi, N. (2010) *The Autism Matrix: The Social Origins of the Autism Epidemic*. Cambridge: Polity.

Frances, A. (2013) *Saving Normal: An Insider's Revolt against Out-Of-Control Psychiatric Diagnosis, DSM-5, Big Pharma, and the Medicalization of Ordinary Life*. New York: Harper Collins.

Gatto, J. T. (2002) *Dumbing Us Down: The Hidden Curriculum of Compulsory Schooling* (rev. ed.). Gabriola Island: New Society Publishers.

Graham, L. J. (2008) 'From ABCs to ADHD: The Role of Schooling in the Construction of Behaviour Disorder and Production of Disorderly Objects', *International Journal of Inclusive Education*, 12(1): 7–33.

Porter, R. (1997) *The Greatest Benefit to Mankind: A Medical History of Humanity*. New York: Norton.

Rafalovich, A. (2004) *Framing ADHD Children: A Critical Examination of the History, Discourse, and Everyday Experience of Attention Deficit/Hyperactivity Disorder*. Lanham, MD: Lexington Books.

Roberts, R. (2015) *Psychology and Capitalism: The Manipulation of Mind.* Alresford: Zero Books.

Rose, N. (1999) *Governing the Soul: The Shaping of the Private Self* (2nd ed.). London: Free Association Books.

Rose, N. (2006) 'Disorders Without Borders? The Expanding Scope of Psychiatric Practice', *BioSocieties*, 1(4): 465–484.

Saul, R. (2014) *ADHD Does Not Exist: The Truth about Attention Deficit and Hyperactivity Disorder*. New York: HarperCollins.

Scull, A. (1993) *The Most Solitary of Afflictions: Madness and Society in Britain, 1700–1900*. New Haven: Yale University Press.

Szasz, T. S. (1997) *The Manufacture of Madness: A Comparative Study of the Inquisition and the Mental Health Movement* (rev. ed.). Syracuse, NY: Syracuse University Press.

Timimi, S. (2008) 'Children's Mental Health and the Global Market: An Ecological Analysis', in Cohen, C. I., and Timimi, S. (Eds.), *Liberatory Psychiatry: Philosophy, Politics, and Mental Health* (pp. 163–182). Cambridge: Cambridge University Press.

Timimi, S. (2009) 'Why Diagnosis of ADHD has Increased so Rapidly in the West: A Cultural Perspective', in Timimi, S., and Leo, J. (Eds.), *Rethinking ADHD: From Brain to Culture* (pp. 133–159). Houndmills, Basingstoke: Palgrave Macmillan.

Whitaker, R., and Cosgrove, L. (2015) *Psychiatry Under the Influence: Institutional Corruption, Social Injury, and Prescriptions for Reform.* New York: Palgrave Macmillan.

Wilkinson, R., and Pickett, K. (2010) *The Spirit Level: Why Equality is Better for Everyone* (rev. ed.). London: Penguin.

6

Women: Reproducing Patriarchal Relations

In the previous chapter I discussed psychiatry's increasing involvement in the surveillance and pathologisation of young people as a strategy for reinforcing the economic and ideological prerogatives of capitalism. The expansion of the psy-professions' interest in this group dwarfs all other areas of concern though, as noted, it only gained real pace with deinstitutionalisation and the rise of neoliberalism. Women, in comparison, have been a focus for systematic psychiatric labelling and oppression for a much longer period of time. Arguably, of all disadvantaged groups, females have been (and remain) psychiatry's real obsession and those most devastated by the medical gaze; so much so that dominant ideas on "mental illness" have often been embodied in the dominant ideals of femininity and the female form. This has been illustrated by Showalter (1985: 1–3) in her discussion of Tony Robert-Fleury's 1887 painting *Pinel Freeing the Insane*. The previously discussed landmark in the formal beginnings of psychiatry with Pinel removing the chains of the insane in Paris in 1793 (Chap. 2) is depicted by the artist as the dominance of (male) rationality and science over (female) irrationality and "nature." In Showalter's (1985: 3) words,

B.M.Z. Cohen, *Psychiatric Hegemony*,
DOI 10.1057/978-1-137-46051-6_6

> [T]he irrationality Pinel frees from its fetters is … visually translated into its most recognisable sign: the beautiful woman, whose disordered body and mind are exposed—and opposed—to the scrutiny of the man who has the authority to unchain her.

It is an oppressive relationship that has endured with the development of the psychiatric profession over the past 200 years. For example, Chesler (2005: 1) more recently stated of her psychoanalytical training in the 1960s and 1970s that "we were taught to view women as somehow naturally mentally ill. Women were hysterics (*hysteros*, the womb), malingerers, child-like, manipulative, either cold or smothering as mothers, and driven to excess by their hormones." As will be recounted in this chapter, the patriarchal ideology within the psy-professions has only intensified over time. The following excerpt from the diagnostic features for histrionic personality disorder (HPD) (American Psychiatric Association 2013: 667), for example, typifies the view of women within the contemporary psychiatric discourse:

> They are overly concerned with impressing others by their appearance and expend an excessive amount of time, energy, and money on clothes and grooming. They may "fish for compliments" regarding appearance and may be easily and excessively upset by a critical comment about how they look or by a photograph that they regard as unflattering.

Women have outnumbered men as psychiatric patients since the mid-nineteenth century and, as Ussher (2011: 1) states, they have been, "more likely to receive psychiatric 'treatment,' ranging from hospitalisation in asylum, accompanied by restraint, electro-convulsive therapy (ECT) and psychosurgery, to psychological therapy and psychotropic drug treatments today."

The history of the psy-professions' pathologisation and abuse of women for being women is deeply disturbing and should shame even the most ardent supporters of the mental health experts. In the name of science and progress, the mental health system has sought to control almost all aspects of women's experiences, emotions, and behaviour through physical and moral interventions. Chesler (2005: 218) notes, for example, that many women were incarcerated in asylums for making claims of sexual abuse against their family, mothering "illegitimate" children, or for "suspected lesbianism." Further, Masson (1986) compiled a collection of highly authoritative psychiatric articles on women from the nineteenth century to vividly demonstrate that acts of physical constraint, rape, torture, and female castration by the profession were all justified as appropriate (if not mandatory) treatment for women who questioned or defied their place in Victorian society. The discussion in this chapter, however, is concerned specifically with explaining the central reasons for previous female oppression by the psy-professions as well as the continuation and expansion in neoliberal society of what Ehrenreich and English (2011) have called the "sexist ideology" of medical professionals. As none of the mental disorders in the DSM with which women have been labelled have validity (Chap. 1), psychiatric interventions cannot be argued to be concerned with the care and treatment of any real distress that women may experience. Instead, we need to understand such institutional interventions within the broader context of structural gender inequalities in capitalist society. As Penfold and Walker (1983: vi) have summated, "[p]sychiatry is an institution in a society in which women are oppressed [and it] plays a specific role in that oppression." A critical understanding of psychiatry's focus on women, gender roles, and deviance can only be fully understood through a thorough assessment of the structural determinants of the division of labour in capitalist society which has devalued female roles and confined women to the status of second-class citizens. This analysis necessitates an investigation of patriarchal forms of domination and the intersectionality with the relations of production—something that has concerned a host of critical feminist scholars since the advent of second wave feminism in the late 1960s. My argument here is that while an examination of the psychiatric profession clearly demonstrates that it continues to be an institution of patriarchal power, the distinctive form that structures this oppression is determined by the needs of capital (such as the requirement for paid and unpaid labour, the reproduction of the labour force, the necessity to suppress working-class resistance, and the normalisation of gender roles in industrial society as "natural," equitable, and common sense). Thus, the critical analysis outlined here follows in the spirit of Donna Haraway (1978: 25) who has succinctly argued that "[t]he biosocial sciences have not simply been sexist mirrors of our own social world. They have also been tools in the reproduction of that world, both in supplying legitimating ideologies and in enhancing material power."

The section that follows discusses how the traditional family structure of agrarian society was fundamentally disrupted by industrialisation and eventuated in the gendered division of labour that demarcated the "private" and "public" spheres of life which, in a slightly adapted form, remain today. Psychiatrists become increasingly important throughout the industrial period as initially incarcerators of deviant working-class women and then as moral enforcers of gender roles, "respectable femininity," and the sanctity of the family. In this way, the institution of psychiatry takes over the moral role previously performed by religion in feudal society. This socio-historical analysis is followed by specific case studies on the diagnoses of hysteria and borderline personality disorder (BPD) to illustrate in detail how psychiatric hegemony serves to regulate prescribed gender roles in capitalist society.

The Division of Labour, Gender Roles, and the Rise of Biological Theory

The moral role that psychiatry plays in enforcing strict gender norms on women is most clearly seen in the development of the profession with the emergence of industrial society in the nineteenth century. As the centre of their developing claims to an expertise on the mad, by the 1850s the asylum is overpopulated with groups of deviant females including single mothers, vagrant and elderly women, and those of supposed "low morals" or low "intelligence." Russell (1995: 13) agrees that during this period, "the basis for committal … was blatantly moral, centring around the notion of dangerousness or relating to social misfits." As a reflection of the expected female role as subservient mother, wife, and carer in Victorian society, drinking, dancing, or even having a political opinion were all potential grounds for psychiatric incarceration (Russell: 1995: 13). The confinement of these mainly working-class women in asylums becomes the backbone of institutional and scientific development of the psychiatric discipline, and the overrepresentation in asylums then provides justification for its focus on mental disease as a distinctive "female malady" (Showalter 1985).

However, mental disorder was not in fact women's problem, rather the shifts in societal relations caused by industrialisation were. Previously, the patriarchal order in agrarian society had demarcated certain forms of work and organisation as the specific domain of women. This included the care and management of livestock and garden and household produce, as well as the acquiring of health and care skills required for raising children and nursing the sick in the family and the local community (Ehrenreich and English 2005: 10–11; see also Hartmann 1976: 148). While women were governed more explicitly by patriarchal rule in the form of the male head of the household—and the ideology of preordained submissiveness of women to men by the church and the state—there was no separation between the biological and economic spheres of production, centring as it did on direct survival and subsistence of the family rather than the production of surplus value for the market. With the emergence of industrial society these old patterns of living are destroyed and, with them, the traditional roles of men and women. As Ehrenreich and English (2005: 12–13) note of this fundamental change,

> When production entered the factory, the household was left with only the most personal biological activities—eating, sex, sleeping, the care of small children, and (until the rise of institutional medicine) birth and dying and the care of the sick and aged. Life would now be experienced as divided into two distinct spheres: a "public" sphere of endeavor governed ultimately by the Market; and a "private" sphere of intimate relationships and individual biological existence.

A more immediate effect brought about by changes in the mode of production from the farm to the factory is the breakdown of the traditional household structure in rural communities; a situation which had a particularly detrimental impact on women. As Russell (1995: 11) notes, it was primarily men who left in search of work in the cities, leaving women vulnerable to single motherhood and vagrancy (respectively, grounds for psychiatric incarceration in nineteenth century England and France). In England, groups of poor and sick women were incarcerated first in workhouses, hospitals, and prisons, and then, with the Lunatics Act of 1845, moved to the burgeoning public asylums (Showalter 1985: 52). This concentration of deviant groups of women within asylums justified a growing fashion in medicine and related sciences for explaining mental pathology in terms of biological degeneracy. In this way, women's deviance is recast in Victorian society as biomedical fact by the new professions. Thus, Ehrenreich and English (2011: 36) have argued that it is with the changes from agricultural to industrial society that we witness, "a pronounced shift from a religious to a biomedical rationale for sexism." Primarily, labelling the poor, disabled, sick, criminal, and dispossessed as "mad" served to manage deviant populations more efficiently in a society where work and production had become highly rationalised. Employment was redefined as a rational and moral choice under industrial conditions, and those who could not or would not meet the demands of the market needed closely supervised management in the new institutions for the deviant—namely, the prison, the poorhouse, the hospital, and the asylum.

The growth in female populations in asylums across Europe and America in the nineteenth century was theorised by psychiatrists under the new medical framework of biological science. Justifications for sex discrimination based on the old ideas of the preordained existence of men and women were no longer adequate within a modern society centred on the principles of science and rationality. If there were differences between men and women in the new order, it would have to be scientifically demonstrated and proven. That proof, argued medicine, could be found in the inherent differences in the biological makeup of men and women. Specifically, it was theorised that the biological functions associated with reproduction left women physically and mentally weaker than men, and more prone to insanity and other forms of disease. As Showalter (1985: 55) confers, the "theories of female insanity were specifically and confidently linked to the biological crisis of the female life cycle—puberty, pregnancy, childbirth, menopause—during which the mind would be weakened and the symptoms of insanity might emerge." Medical theories of female biology were thus used as scientific legitimation for the emerging division of labour in industrial society.

Unchained from the land and the old patriarchal order, industrial society offered women potential new freedoms, yet the factory system robbed women of their traditional forms of production and over time forced them into the highly regulated domestic sphere of the home (Ehrenreich and English 2005: 17). The rationalised family structure for industrial towns and cities required a fulltime unpaid worker in the home who could reproduce the future labour force, take care of the young, old and sick in the immediate family, and create a supportive environment for the paid worker who was now employed outside of the family unit. This particular division of labour inside and outside the home was embedded in new forms of patriarchal oppression predicated on redefining "productive labour" as that referring only to the waged labour of the public sphere. As Kynaston (1996: 224) explains, "[t]asks will be labelled productive or unproductive, and will be paid or unpaid, depending upon whether they are performed in the capitalist workplace or in the home." The private sphere of the home—separated from the more "valued" but harsher marketplace—becomes a refuge; in Ehrenreich and English's (2005: 14) words,

> private life now takes on a sentimental appeal in proportion to the coldness and impersonality of the "outside" world. [Men] look to the home to fulfill both the bodily needs denied at the workplace, and the human solidarity forbidden in the Market.

Biological theories served to justify this division of labour and scientifically condemn women to less private and public power than men. The gender divisions created and maintained within industrial society are then rationalised through patriarchal institutions such as medicine as common sense notions of what men and women truly are. For example, the German zoologist Karl Ernst von Baer (cited in Libbon 2007: 85) argued,

> In man, the mind prevails—in woman, the emotions. The former takes pleasure in the production of thoughts, the latter in the mental reception of feelings. Man's aspirations are directed outwards towards a broader sphere; woman cares for the narrower circle of the family. Man's purpose is creative; woman's essence is conservative and protective. Knowledge and

> ideas guide the will of man; in the action of woman sentiment prevails over thinking and guides her though in a less clearly conscious manner.

As Fraad et al. (1989: 15) remark, pervasive ever since in western society is the gendered conceptions of "housework and childrearing as 'natural' or 'preferred' vocations for females, while other kinds of labor performed outside the home are more 'natural' or 'preferred' for males." Throughout the nineteenth century scientists produced evidence—such as anatomical studies showing thinner ligaments, smaller skulls, and generally "weaker" bodies of the female—which they argued could demonstrate exactly why women are biologically and intellectually inferior to men and therefore more appropriately assigned to reproductive and domestic duties (Libbon 2007: 82). Simultaneously, such research becomes a useful justification for paying what remains of the working population of women less and restricting their labour participation to supporting roles (including within the asylum system itself, where Showalter (1985: 52–53) notes that the number of women in senior attendant roles declined as the number of female inmates increased).

Libbon (2007: 86–87) highlights that the verve of patriarchal science to prove sex role differentiation throughout the nineteenth century correlates with the increasing dissatisfaction and protest by women against such gender demarcations. As the century progresses, the "woman question" becomes a popular topic of debate across Europe and America, and the developing profession of psychiatry comes to play a more prominent role in reinforcing the morality of "appropriate" gender roles. For example, Darwinian psychiatry of the 1870s proclaimed women as less evolved than men due to their physiology; the dominance of the reproductive system meant that the female brain was largely incapacitated, thus women were theorised as "naturally" reliant and submissive to the superior male race (Showalter 1985: 121–125). Psychiatric scholars argued that there was a danger of insanity if women sought to exert additional pressure on the brain through seeking an education or considering political matters. Even the simple activities of writing or reading could be potentially disastrous to a woman's health, as can be seen from the following advice given to prominent feminist writer Charlotte Perkins Gilman (cited in

Ehrenreich and English 2005: 112) by her doctor in the latter part of the nineteenth century:

> Live as domestic a life as possible. Have your child with you all the time ... Lie down an hour after each meal. Have but two hours intellectual life a day. And never touch pen, brush or pencil as long as you live.

Feminists became a prime target for the psychological sciences; such women were theorised as degenerative, sexually deviant and a threat to the "natural order" of the species (Libbon 2007: 86–87). According to the famous sexologist Krafft-Ebing, the dangers for women of abandoning their prescribed sex role were becoming "too masculine" as well as sexually permissive, both of which could be considered as regressive and pathological—symptoms of underlying organic damage to the female body (Libbon 2007: 87). Under the patriarchal ideology of the experts of the mind, mental disorders such as nymphomania, hyperesthesia (a mental illness caused by "oversensitivity"), and hysteria became commonly associated with those women who dared to deviate from the strict confines of Victorian femininity and their ascribed domestic chores. Thus, the dominant discourse on the division of labour and gender roles in industrial society was legitimated and reinforced by the burgeoning psy-professions as normal, common sense, and healthy for society. "Mental breakdown," remarks Showalter (1985: 123), "would come when the women defied their 'nature,' attempted to compete with men instead of serving them, or sought alternatives or even additions to their maternal functions."

The increased labelling and confinement of women as "mad" by psychiatry served to legitimate the needs of capital and patriarchy for subservient and conforming women under the discourse of medical science. Here, we see the development of what would become the hegemonic domination of female populations by psychiatry and its allies—professional groups that have sought to depoliticise the struggle against patriarchal power through medicalising women's bodies and experiences as pathological. As Libbon (2007: 89) summates of psychiatry's success in the nineteenth century,

> Having labelled woman as intrinsically diseased and debauched, experts and laymen alike now took institutional measures to impede any further social or political disruption on her part. Under the guise of "curing" her of her ailments and moreover protecting society in the process, the unruly woman was now forced either into compulsory hospitalization, often with accompanying surgical mutilation, or incarceration. In both instances it was the woman who protested and rallied against male control and regulation of herself and her body who was locked away, sequestered from society, in an effort to compel her to return to … the silent, submissive role man had eked out for her.

Deviant Women and Physical "Treatments"

"Fast forward more than a century," states Ussher (2011: 65), "and many would argue things have not greatly changed." Yet things have changed, and for the worse. The labelling of deviant women as mentally unstable has become more systematic and more sophisticated. So much so that women are now self-policing their own mental states under patriarchal and capitalist ideologies of women's expected roles, duties, and responsibilities in neoliberal society. In the twentieth century, the psy-professions expanded their spheres of influence beyond the institution and the therapist's office, into—among other places—the home, the school, and the workplace. As will be outlined in this section, psychiatry further developed their misogynistic theories and practices on women as part of extending their claims to expertise on the mind, and through modes of "treatment" in the institutional environment, including ECT and psychosurgery. The development of successive editions of the DSM cemented ideas on female pathology as a part of "scientific progress," rather than the enforcement of culturally prescribed gender roles. We shall see that feminised categories of mental disorder in the DSM grow with the decline of psychiatric hospitals and in response to the changing needs for labour in neoliberal society. New drug treatments are developed and explicitly aimed at females who remain unsatisfied with the increasingly complex and demanding nature of their roles as lower-paid workers, primary homemakers, and carers, as well as mothers. As will be illustrated with reference to my textual analysis of each DSM, psychiatric hegemony serves to depoliticise the reality of women's experiences through recasting patriarchal and capitalist oppression as personal distress and individual pathology.

While first wave feminism had achieved significant advances for women in the spheres of education, politics and employment in the late nineteenth and early twentieth centuries, "[b]y the 1920s," notes Showalter (1985: 196), "women found themselves with little progress besides the vote." Though capitalism required more women in the workplace during periods of economic expansion and wartime, women's primary responsibility remained in the home, reproducing the future workers and caring for the family. Psychiatric theories on the female malady adapted to reflect these changing economic and social conditions; now it was argued that meaningful work could potentially make women mentally stronger and less prone to mental illness (Showalter 1985: 195). These evolving psychiatric ideas, however, were tempered by the enforcement of appropriate gender roles along strongly classed lines, whereas middle-class women were patronised by new Freudian ideas in the therapist's office, working-class women were being incarcerated in the still expanding asylum system.

Freud's psychoanalytic theory was—and continues to be—a significant challenge to biomedical psychiatry but not, however, to dominant ideas on gender roles. On the contrary, psychoanalysis was rooted in the same set of patriarchal assumptions on "respectable femininity" which sought to reinforce the home and the family as women's "natural" location. The new psychiatric "treatment" of "therapy" gained momentum particularly during the 1920s and 1930s, with the ultimate purpose of psychoanalysis being to "educate women in therapy to be better wives and mothers" (Penfold and Walker 1983: 90). It is more than coincidence that psychoanalysis became popular in Europe and America at a time when middle-class women continued to feel deeply marginalised despite the gains achieved by first wave feminism. As Horney (cited in Caplan and Cosgrove 2004: xxvi–xxvii) commented in the 1920s of Freud's notion of "penis envy," it was the privileges and power afforded to men that continued to be denied to women which was at issue, not the psychoanalytic delusion that women were at all perturbed at the denial of a penis. Psychoanalysis may have been a radical challenge to the "scientific psychiatry" of Kraepelin and others (Chap. 2), but it was a case of old wine in new bottles for extending the oppressive patriarchal practices of the mental health system.

Restricted to the public setting of the mental hospital, biomedical psychiatry continued to confine greater numbers of deviant working-class women for longer periods of time within their walls. These women included uncooperative housewives, widows, single mothers, those sexually or physically abused by family members or relatives, as well as those women considered in some other way to be immoral, criminal, aggressive, or generally "unfeminine." With the neurotic disorders more likely to be labels used with middle-class women in therapy, hospitalised working-class females were typically labelled as schizophrenic and subjected to the new biomedical "treatments" for insanity including insulin coma therapy, ECT, and psychosurgery (Showalter 1985: 204–205).

The evidence that has since been collected clearly demonstrates the use of such biomedical interventions to punish deviant women and reinforce conformity to the desired feminine gender role. For example, ECT—something Burstow (cited in Ussher 2011: 84) has bluntly described as "state sponsored violence against women"—has been disproportionately inflicted on women. Breggin suggests that this is because women are judged by the mental experts, "to have less need of their brains" (cited in Showalter 1985: 207). The sex role assumptions made by the psychiatric profession that women should be docile and confined to the domestic sphere have made disobedient and aggressive women a particular target for ECT throughout the twentieth century (Showalter 1985: 207). In her own account of being hospitalised in 1961, Janet Frame (cited in Ussher 2011: 83)—one of New Zealand's most celebrated novelists—recalled that ECT was a constant threat for nonconforming and "difficult" women. As a result,

> you learned with earnest dedication to "fit in"; you learned not to cry in company but to smile and pronounce yourself pleased, and to ask from time if you could go home, as proof you were getting better and therefore in no need to be smuggled in the night to Ward Two [for ECT]. You

> learned the chores, to make your bed with the government motto facing the correct way and the corners of the counterpane neatly angled.

While the use of ECT decreased with deinstitutionalisation in the 1970s, it has had a recent revival in the new century with women continuing to be overrepresented in the statistics (Ussher 2011: 83–84). As Ussher has outlined, ECT remains a form of medical control against deviant and resistant wives and mothers in the twenty-first century; ECT can be used as a threat to produce compliance in the patient but, more than this, to “restore women to ‘normal’ marital functioning” (Ussher 2011: 86). Citing Johnstone’s research on experiences of ECT, Ussher (2011: 86) recalls women being told by psychiatric staff that upsetting or worrying their husbands is “not a good thing for a wife to do,” and that the treatment—often resulting in memory loss as well as a fear of repeat treatments—was being given, “for the sake of the family.”

As appropriate to their gender roles in the highly conservative nuclear families of the 1940s and 1950s, the lobotomy promised to return frustrated housewives, hostile mothers, and antagonistic women to the home as more submissive and docile models (Chap. 2). Housewives were considered excellent candidates for the procedure by psychosurgeons because it allowed women to better cope with marriage and family obligations (Showalter 1985: 210). Certainly, in England it has been recorded that the majority of lobotomies carried out were performed on women (Showalter 1985: 209). Such radical interventions further demonstrate psychiatry as an institution of social control, responsible for reinforcing the expected female role through “symbolic episodes of punishment for intellectual ambition, domestic defiance, and sexual autonomy” (Showalter 1985: 210). Such physical treatments were eventually replaced following the introduction of the drug chlorpromazine (marketed as Thorazine in America) in the late 1950s. Chlorpromazine was marketed as the chemical equivalent of a lobotomy (Chap. 2), yet cheaper and—in theory—safer than psychosurgery. Uncooperative women were again targeted for this treatment, a situation which has continued with the rapid growth in drug treatments and the increasing number of psychiatric diagnoses focused on women. As Diamond (2014: 195) has summarised, women seeking help from the mental health system in the twenty-first century remain, "twice as likely [as men] to be given pscyhopharmaceutical drugs."

Neoliberalism and "Feminising" the DSM

Deinstitutionalisation has been bittersweet for women. The successes of second wave feminism in challenging the traditional gender roles of mothers and wives has seen an expansion in the psychiatric surveillance and monitoring of the "new woman" outside of the home. This is witnessed, for example, in the steady increase in the number of "feminised" categories of mental illness in the DSM which problematise the female role, and in which women are typically overrepresented (see Table 6.1).

While still being the primary carer in the home, the demands of neoliberal society for women to engage in the labour market is matched by the increasing variety of ways that the psychiatric discourse has sought to medicalise women's bodies and experiences. The introduction of premenstrual dysphoric disorder (PMDD) to full mental disorder status in the DSM-5, for example, demonstrates the profession's successful pathologisation of menstruation. The "symptoms" of this disorder include a "lack of energy," "specific food cravings," and "physical symptoms such as breast tenderness or swelling, joint or muscle pain, a sensation of 'bloating,' or weight gain" (American Psychiatric Association 2013: 172). As Moynihan and Cassels (2005: 100) wryly note, "[t]he emotional ups and downs preceding your period are no longer a part of normal life—they are now a telltale sign you could have a psychiatric disorder." During the development of the DSM-IV in the early 1990s, Paula Caplan served on the APA committee responsible for reviewing the research evidence for the PMDD category (then titled late luteal phase dysphoric disorder (LLPDD)). She subsequently resigned from the committee on the

Table 6.1 Number of "feminised" diagnostic categories in the DSM, 1952–2013[a]

DSM-I (1952)	DSM-II (1968)	DSM-III (1980)	DSM-III-R (1987)	DSM-IV (1994)	DSM-IV-TR (2000)	DSM-5 (2013)
4	9	19	16	21	25	24

[a]See Appendix C for full diagnostic list.

grounds that there was no empirical evidence for PMDD, stating that instead there were clear social and political dangers in introducing a category so blatantly aimed at pathologising women's bodies (Caplan 1995: 122–167). Despite protests from Caplan and other researchers, the APA still introduced the disorder to the appendices of the DSM-IV. PMDD and its previous incarnations of LLPDD, premenstrual syndrome (PMS), and premenstrual tension (PMT) have been perfect patriarchal designations with which to label women as biologically out of control, a prisoner to their own hormones. For over 80 years this disorder has served to reinforce respectable femininity and police women's complaints associated with their restricted roles in capitalist society. As Chrisler and Caplan (2002: 283) have noted of the construction of PMT in 1931, it "provided a sound, medical (i.e., scientific) reason why women should stay out of the workforce and leave to men any jobs that were available." As the neoliberal equivalent, however, the current variant is more concerned with pathologising the "unproductive" woman. As the DSM-5 (American Psychiatric Association 2013: 172, emphasis added) explicitly states, "[t]he symptoms [of PMDD] are associated with clinically significant distress or interference with work, school, usual social activities, or relationships with others (e.g., avoidance of social activities; *decreased productivity and efficiency at work, school, or home*)."

Parker (2007: 69–70) reminds us that the neoliberal workplace has become increasingly "feminised" with the growth in service sector and leisure industries, and the greater focus on employee's interpersonal and "emotional" skills in areas such as business, commerce, and marketing. Female participation in the US labour force has increased from less than a third in the 1940s to 57 per cent currently (the comparative rate for males is 70 per cent) (U.S. Bureau of Labor Statistics 2014: 1), with the figures for most European countries being slightly higher (The Globalist 2015). Women have also become more visible in senior management roles, with over 20 per cent of these positions now filled globally by females (Grant Thornton 2012). Unchained from the traditional sites of female labour and empowered by the economic freedoms of the marketplace, young women would now appear to be the emancipated versions that their mothers had dreamed of and fought for with second wave feminism. However, compared to men, women remain poorly paid in less secure jobs, are still grossly underrepresented in management positions, and continue to undertake the majority of the housework and domestic responsibilities (The Globe and Mail 2013; Grant Thornton 2012; U.S. Bureau of Labor Statistics 2014: 2–3).

The psy-professions have become increasingly important in the management of these changing gender roles, and in promoting the ideology of the "normal" feminine subject who is constantly self-monitoring her own behaviour and emotions. This can be seen, for instance, in the changes in the psychiatric discourse on gender and women with each DSM. Contrary to what common sense might suggest about medicine moving away from the sexist clichés of the female form found in textbooks on pathology 50 years ago, the psychiatric profession has actually sought to reinstate and multiply their focus on aspects of the "feminine" within the DSM, with increased references to hormones, physical appearance, housework, the family, childbirth, and (predominantly female) sexuality within their diagnostic creations (see Table 6.2). The proliferation of such wording and phasing in each DSM as neoliberalism has progressed—especially the total count increase witnessed with DSM-III, DSM-IV, and DSM-5—is evidence of the increasing usefulness of psychiatric discourse as a means of ideological control of female behaviour, both policing the boundaries of acceptable gender roles as well as reinforcing heteronormativity.

Following the physical "treatments" that the institution used to assert patriarchal authority over women by coercive means, the ideological function of psychiatry has expanded with the merging of biomedicine and neoliberalism (see, e.g., Moncrieff 2008). Explicitly, the growth in psychopharmaceuticals since the 1970s has succeeded in promoting self-monitoring practices and potential coping mechanisms for the multiple roles now demanded of women. In the advertising of antidepressants, for example, females are dominantly portrayed as hindered by their own biology; "emancipation" for women in neoliberal society is therefore only possible by self-diagnosing and self-medicating behaviour (Ussher 2011: 88–91). "Tapping into a post-feminist neoliberal discourse of equality," remarks Ussher (2011: 90) of such adverts, "women are portrayed as being able to work productively alongside men, as long as they are liberated from hormonal or mood fluctuations." As with

Table 6.2 Number of gender-related words/phrases in the DSM, 1952–2013[a]

Word/phrase	DSM-I (1952)	DSM-II (1968)	DSM-III (1980)	DSM-III-R (1987)	DSM-IV (1994)	DSM-IV-TR (2000)	DSM-5 (2013)
Abortion	0	7	1	1	1	1	1
Eating disorder	0	0	19	20	65	56	130
Family	26	1	123	97	157	164	193
Female	24	9	77	195	298	287	385
Feminine/ty	0	0	6	9	10	12	9
Gender/ed/identity/disorder/dysphoria	0	0	46	84	269	306	567
Home/housework	2	2	59	80	92	96	109
Hormone/s/al	1	3	2	8	11	13	20
Hysteria/ical	27	19	48	29	2	0	0
Menopause/al	1	1	2	4	10	11	9
Menstrual/tion/cycle/menses	2	2	7	26	87	65	19
Obese/ity	1	1	7	8	13	12	68
Over/under/weight	3	1	56	82	172	171	235
Physical/appearance	0	0	1	3	6	8	18
Pregnant/cy/childbirth	0	25	21	22	17	21	47
Sexual/ity	18	24	565	643	948	919	1166
Woman/en	0	0	44	28	85	141	120
Total count	105	94	1084	1339	2243	2283	3096

[a]See Appendix A for methodology

the increasing range of feminised mental illness labels, antidepressants would appear to offer women "freedom" from the increasing demands of neoliberal society; a view articulated in Peter Kramer's book *Listening to Prozac* (1994) when the psychiatrist argues that selective serotonin reuptake inhibitors (SSRIs) can be understood as "feminist" solutions to the realities of women's current economic and social situation. Taking antidepressants, he suggests, can increase confidence and energy levels while allowing women to become "less serious" about family circumstances such as finding a life partner or dealing with marital stress (cited in Tseris and Cohen 2016: 422). In this way, psychiatric hegemony successfully depoliticises continuing gender inequalities in capitalist society through the promotion of technologies of self-governance rather than collective political action. The following section demonstrates the continuity of the psy-professional surveillance of women from the construction of hysteria in the nineteenth century to the current DSM-5 equivalent of BPD.

Case Studies: Hysteria and Borderline Personality Disorder

Psychiatry's policing of femininity within industrial society has played a key role in maintaining patriarchal power. Validity for the knowledge claims and practices of the mental health system has been achieved on the basis of enforcing the division of labour through the construction of mental illness labels which reinforce dominant gender roles and punish deviations from them. Far from vanishing in the twenty-first century, the diagnosis of hysteria has in fact fragmented and morphed into many more "feminised" categories of pathology which can be found in the DSM-5 today. As some psy-professionals have already argued (see, e.g., Becker 1997: 77; Goldstein 1982: 211), these categories of mental illness need to be considered as "waste basket" diagnoses; they are categories into which any and every woman can be placed as necessary for the maintenance of male dominance. This is as true for the current BPD label as it was for the classic category of hysteria.

It does not happen very often, but when a category of mental illness is removed from the DSM there are always those psychiatrists that mourn its passing into history. Perhaps this is less so with the blatant pro-slavery category of drapetomania (Chap. 7) and the inherent homophobia of including homosexuality in the DSM-I and the DSM-II, but there are still calls for hysteria to be considered a valid mental illness today (see, e.g., Stone et al. 2008). The good news for these psychiatrists is that the spirit of hysteria remains in many other DSM-5 categories. As Micale (1993: 525) explains of what has happened to the diagnosis, it "lacked a strong etiological theory to hold it together," so instead the hysteria classification has been, "effectively broken down into its constituent symptomatological parts, which were then reassembled in new combinations and distributed to many other medical categories." We should not be surprised: as a racialised category of mental disorder, drapetomania morphed into schizophrenia and "cannabis psychosis" (Chap. 7), homosexuality became a part of gender identity disorder (GID) and, more recently, gender dysphoria (GD). Once created, psychiatric diagnoses never really disappear but are instead recycled into many more categories of mental illness.

Despite the eventual disappearance of the hysteria diagnosis in the mid-twentieth century, official historians of psychiatry remain keen to evoke the label as a timeless—though often misunderstood—part of human experience. After all, the term was used in the ancient civilisations of Egypt and Greece to denote physical pathology in women resulting from the movement of the womb (Veith 1970: 10). Thus, states Shorter (1997: 22), such mental pathologies, "have accompanied humankind," and "have always been with us." Yet many of the nineteenth century physicians who believed in the reality of the disorder conceded that the hysteria classification was a chaotic mess of contrasting and overlapping behaviours and symptoms. This included the inventor of the famous "rest cure" for the disorder, Silas Weir Mitchell, who often referred to the diagnosis as "mysteria" (Scull 2009: 6–7). In contrast, what a sociocultural analysis of hysteria more closely identifies is the ongoing moral persecution of women by medicine, as Allison and Roberts (1994: 239) remark,

> Throughout the history of medicine from the early Greeks up to the end of the nineteenth century, the definition and diagnosis of hysteria had a function similar to that found in the persecution of witchcraft: it sought to eradicate the outbursts of nonconforming and emotionally threatening conduct of women.

Consequently, summates Gibson (2004: 201), "the diagnosis has served the status quo from its politically motivated construction to its socially constructed present."

The appropriation of the hysteria label by the emerging psychiatric profession served a number of specific purposes in the nineteenth century. Firstly, it aided the legitimisation of the profession with other branches of scientific medicine through furthering biological explanations for the pathology (in this case, the unwarranted behaviour of the uterus). Secondly, the diagnosis gave a historically credible lineage which could be traced all the way back to Hippocrates, the "father of western medicine" (Allison and Roberts 1994: 243). Thus, the classification gave psychiatric science a "progressive" medical narrative to further legitimate their expanding activities. Thirdly, increased protests against the constraints on the female role could be reconstituted as an organic mental disorder over which women had little control (Russell 1995: 25); in this way, social and political threats to the contemporary patriarchal order became increasingly seen as evidence of the irrationality and "hysterical" proclivity of women. As Showalter (1985: 145) maintains, of all the nervous disorders with which women were labelled, "hysteria was the most strongly identified with the feminist movement." Above all, psychiatry's success was tied to the labelling of resistant women as hysterical, which in turn supported the status quo of industrial capitalism; women were required to work and perform in the supportive domestic sphere, and deviations from their prescribed roles as dutiful wives, mothers, and carers would be punished.

Hysteria was originally conceptualised by Hippocrates as a physical disorder caused by the wandering of the uterus to different parts of the body. This was hypothesised as leading to a great number of disorders and disturbances, as Allison and Roberts (1994: 242, emphasis original) explain,

> In certain cases, the upward movement of the uterus (the *hystera*) would cause great irritation and pain in the pelvis; in other cases, it moved directly into the throat, creating a sensation of strangulation caused by the imaginary sensation of a lump in the throat (*globus hystericus*); in still others, it might cause flushing, paralysis, seizures, violent headaches, fits of sobbing, etc.

Virgins, widows, and spinsters were considered as more susceptible to the affliction due to the "drying out" of the uterus (Allison and Roberts 1994: 242). The cure for hysteria therefore suggested by Hippocrates was "marriage, remarriage, and intercourse" (Allison and Roberts 1994: 243). Two millennia later, psychiatric physicians hypothesised the aetiology and treatment of hysteria in a strikingly similar manner: women remained prisoners of their biology and vulnerable to mental disease if they should venture beyond the domestic sphere, overexertion caused by such pursuits as education or employment could cause the womb to yet again wander. A conception of women as physically and mentally weak as symbolised by the hysteria label, notes Cayleff (1988: 1202), both explained and reinforced the ideological justification of women as "naturally" more suited for childbearing and emotional work within the home. Those women of an independent or rebellious nature were particularly at risk of the disorder, as one gynaecologist (cited in Smith-Rosenberg and Rosenberg 1973: 341) complained of the college-educated female in 1901,

> She may be highly cultured and accomplished and shine in society, but her future husband will discover too late that he has married a large outfit of headaches, backaches and spine aches, instead of a woman fitted to take up the duties of life.

Likewise, Showalter (1985: 145) cites F.C. Skey's observations of his hysterical patients in 1866 as, "exhibiting more than usual force and decision of character, of strong resolution, fearless of character." The hysteria label therefore reinforced dominant sex roles by prescribing the idea of home life as the healthy and "natural" place for women. Therapeutic solutions recommended by psychiatry for women were naturally located in the home—through marriage, having a child, responding positively to their husband's sexual advances, as well as being more involved in domestic chores and less in intellectual activities. For example, Smith-Rosenberg and Rosenberg (1973: 341) note that the involvement in house-cleaning activities was recommended for the "servant-coddled American girl" who might otherwise fall prey to hysteria. Those so labelled as hysterics were often considered by psychiatrists as difficult to treat and "fakers, self-indulgent, undisciplined, and morally weak" women who were failing in their prescribed duties as middle-class wives and mothers (Jimenez 1997: 157).

As the struggle for women's rights increased in the latter decades of the nineteenth century, the hysteria label was increasingly utilised as a catch-all mental disease for any woman exhibiting behaviour considered as troublesome and a threat to the tightly constructed Victorian sex roles. Psychiatry could label women as hysterical for being "unfeminine" and overaggressive if they had sympathies for the suffrage movement or failed to have children at their husband's request or, in contrast, for being "over-sensitive" and emotional, refusing to eat or keep the home in order, being constantly tired, or prone to crying. In short, the hysteria label could be applied to any aspect of female behaviour, and as Ussher (2011: 9) states, was eventually, "linked to the essence of femininity itself." By the turn of the century, the validity of the diagnosis was beginning to be questioned within the profession as some physicians disparagingly referred to it as the "wastebasket of medicine" (Lesegne, cited in Ussher 2011: 10). The introduction of Freud and Breuer's famous work on the aetiology of hysteria undermined the somatic (physical or biological) foundation for the disorder, instead emphasising the supposed "sexual neurosis" of women suffering from "classic hysteria" (Allison and Roberts 1994: 253). Sexual trauma—firstly theorised as real, but then hastily altered by Freud to imagined (see Masson 1992)—rather than organic predisposition could more precisely explain such women's complex array of neurotic symptoms. Even if sexual neurosis appeared at first to be absent from female complaints, Freud believed that with enough therapy the anxieties of, for example, being a virgin, being over- or under-aroused by men, or wanting to be loved, would eventually surface. In this way, Freud's work continued the psychiatric pathologisation of women but with a more distinct framing of "female problems" as sexual in nature (Allison and Roberts 1994: 255). Ironically, as Allison and Roberts (1994: 257–8) recall, this narrowing of the hysteria diagnosis led to its virtual disappearance in the early twentieth century, and its replacement by many more varieties of neuroses, phobias, and other personality disorders which would eventually find their way into the DSM.

Reflecting the conservative values of post-war society and capitalism's need to remove women from the factories and return to the home, the DSM-I (American Psychiatric Association 1952) retained a plethora of hysteria diagnoses, while the DSM-II (American Psychiatric Association 1968: 43) reinforced the gender-specific nature of the "hysterical personality (histrionic personality disorder)" classification as follows:

> These behavior patterns are characterized by excitability, emotional instability, over-reactivity, and self-dramatization. This self-dramatization is always attention-seeking and often seductive, whether or not the patient is aware of its purpose. These personalities are also immature, self-centered, often vain, and usually dependent on others.

However, the results of second wave feminism in the 1960s and 1970s, along with changes in the composition of the workforce and emergent neoliberal policies, led to altered expectations of gender roles within western society. Women remained the primary caregiver and homemaker, yet also became increasingly visible in the public sphere and significant in the world of work. The new woman was independent, decisive, and single minded. She had control of her own reproductive capabilities and demanded respect and equal rights to men in all spheres of life. In sum, the modern woman was a clear threat to patriarchal authority and capitalism's need for future workers and a reserve army of labour. Institutions of civil society in the late twentieth century were, thus, responsible for reinforcing gender differences and demarcating sex roles as natural while fundamentally progressive. As Jimenez (1997: 161) puts it, "[t]he apparent permanence of the changes in gender roles that followed the feminist movement and other social changes of the 1960s and 1970s led to a revision of psychiatric norms regarding appropriate behavior for women." The response of western psychiatry as represented by the APA's DSM-III (American Psychiatric Association 1980) was to update their conceptions of appropriate gender roles, portraying the modern woman as increasingly prone to mental illness due to a combination of the increased pressures from her multiple roles in society, as well as her abandonment of the home and the family as her "natural" environment. Consequently, the "hysterical personality" diagnosis was renamed histrionic personality disorder (HPD), a classification which remains in the DSM to this day. As Jimenez (1997: 158) notes, the symptoms of this modern diagnosis bore a striking similarity to those which psychiatrists offered for the nineteenth century "hysteric." The sufferer of HPD was "[e]ssentially a caricature of exaggerated femininity," with symptoms suggesting childlike, manipulative, vain, excitable, immature, and overdramatic behaviour. (Meanwhile, the version of HPD in the DSM-5 reads like a thinly veiled misogynist rant against a female partner who—in the words of the APA—often acts out the role of either "victim" or "princess" in their relationship with others (APA 2013: 668)).

As a significant "feminised" category of mental illness, however, HPD was superseded in the DSM-III by the introduction of the controversial BPD, a label which has been increasingly applied to women, with around 75 per cent of all cases estimated to be female (Becker 1997: xxii–xxiii). Seen as a milder form of schizophrenia and lying on the "borderline" between neuroses and psychoses, the concept has been used in psychiatry since 1938 (Decker 2013: 196). Like other personality disorders, BPD has a notoriously low reliability level even by the generally poor standards of the DSM, and even within the profession is considered by many as yet another "wastebasket" category (though as Bourne (2011: 76) ruefully remarks, the ambiguity of such personality disorders makes them particularly useful in policing deviance in the new century). One member of the DSM-III task force stated at the time of constructing BPD that "in my opinion, the borderline syndrome stands for everything that is wrong with psychiatry [and] the category should be eliminated" (cited in Decker 2013:199). The chair of the task force, Robert Spitzer, admitted with the publication of DSM-III that BPD was only included in the manual due to pressures from psychoanalytically oriented clinicians who found it useful in their practices (Spitzer 1980: 31–32). Such practices have been documented by Luhrmann (2000: 113) who describes psychiatrists' typical view of the BPD patient as "an angry, difficult woman—almost always a woman—given to intense, unstable relationships and a tendency to make suicide attempts as a call for help." Bearing significant similarities to the feelings of nineteenth century psychiatrists towards hysterics, Luhrmann's (2000: 115) study reveals psychiatrists' revulsion of those they label with a personality disorder: they are "patients you don't like, don't trust, don't want … One of the reasons you dislike them is an expungable sense that they are morally at fault because they choose to be different." Becker (1997: xv) reinforces this general view of the BPD label when she states that "[t]here is no other diagnosis currently in use that has the intense pejorative connotations that have been attached to the borderline personality disorder diagnosis." A bitter irony for those labelled with BPD is that many are known to have experienced sexual abuse in childhood (Ussher 2011: 81), something they share in common with many of those Freud labelled as hysterical a century earlier; a psychiatric pattern of depoliticising sexual abuse by ignoring the (usually) male perpetrator, and instead pathologising the survival mechanisms of the victim as abnormal (Caplan 1995: 237).

By the mid-1980s, the hysteria diagnosis had disappeared from the clinical setting while BPD had become the most commonly diagnosed personality disorder (Bourne 2011: 76). BPD is now the most important label which psychiatric hegemony invokes to serve capital and patriarchy through monitoring and controlling the modern woman, reinforcing expected gender roles within the more fluid, neoliberal environment. Nevertheless, as Jimenez (1997: 163, emphasis added) reminds us, the historical continuity from hysteria to BPD is clear:

> Both diagnoses delimit appropriate behavior for women, and many of the criteria are stereotypically feminine. What distinguishes borderline personality disorder from hysteria is the inclusion of anger and other aggressive characteristics, such as shoplifting, reckless driving, and substance abuse. *If the hysteric was a damaged woman, the borderline woman is a dangerous one.*

The overemotional, needy housewife of the nineteenth century had been replaced at the end of the twentieth century by Glenn Close in the film *Fatal Attraction* (1987)—an out of control, irrational, aggressive (if unknowing) victim of women's liberation. As the DSM-5 (American Psychiatric Association 2013: 664) states of the BPD sufferer,

> Easily bored, they may constantly seek something to do. Individuals with this disorder frequently express inappropriate, intense anger or have difficulty controlling their anger ... They may display extreme sarcasm, enduring bitterness, or verbal outbursts. The anger is often elicited when a caregiver or lover is seen as neglectful, withholding, uncaring, or abandoning. Such expressions of anger are often followed by shame and guilt and contribute to the feeling they have of being evil.

BPD asserts a moral code on the neoliberal woman, defining the limits of her independence in line with dominant, expected gender roles in the twenty-first century. Thus, the introduction of such categories to the DSM is far from accidental. In contrast, Jimenez (1997: 166–167) insightfully states,

> It was related to the social and cultural gains women achieved in the 1970s, when many middle-class women moved into the public sphere, increasing their independence and reshuffling gender roles. These personality disorders define the mentally healthy woman as one who is renewed and energized by social change and no longer dependent on men, but neither angry nor aggressive. According to the criteria, a woman who is mentally healthy restrains her sexuality and does not use her new powers to manipulate men. Together, these diagnoses demonstrate psychiatry's ability not only to respond to changes in gender-role arrangements, but to limit their impact.

Personality disorders such as BPD serve as the latest versions of supposed scientifically valid medical classifications with which to police and control women's behaviour in neoliberal society. As Ussher (2011: 81) has reiterated, it is a historically persistent form of social control of women that powerful forces in society have considered deviant:

> As the outspoken, difficult woman of the sixteenth century was castigated as a witch, and the same woman in the nineteenth century a hysteric, in the late twentieth and twenty-first centuries, she is described as "borderline." All are stigmatising labels. All are irrevocably tied to what it means to be a "woman" at a particular point in history.

Summary

From nymphomania to PMDD, the labelling of women as mentally disordered has been a successful mechanism through which psy-professionals have gained prestige and power in capitalist society. As I have discussed in this chapter, psychiatry has always been an institution of patriarchal power, responsible for reinforcing gender roles as natural and common sense while pathologising any potential deviations from these. Though "feminised" diagnoses lack validity, they have served to support the dominant economic and ideological prerogatives for compliant mothers, wives, carers, and (increasingly) workers. Unlike other patriarchal institutions, however, psychiatrists and allied professions have had the advantage of being able to transform the lived conditions, experiences, and behaviour of women into medical symptoms of pathology. As Jimenez (1997: 171) has stated of this process of medicalisation, "[p]sychiatry's ideas about appropriate gender-role behavior are hardly unique. What is unique is its role in the social construction of disease: Through the reification of its diagnostic system, psychiatry translates gender ideologies into definable codes for women's behavior." In neoliberal society, the demands on women have only increased and, with them, the number of psychiatric labels which can be applied to those who fail to be productive, self-regulating individuals. Thus, as the psychiatric discourse has reached hegemonic status, the surveillance of the female has continued to be a significant part of psy-professional activity. In this chapter I included discussion of the ways in which social and political protest by women has been pathologised by the mental health experts, the following chapter explores more general issues of dissent and collective resistance to capitalism and, in doing so, the—symbolically and physically—violent psychiatric responses to these.

Bibliography

Allison, D. B., and Roberts, M. S. (1994) 'On Constructing the Disorder of Hysteria', *Journal of Medicine and Philosophy*, 19(3): 239–259.

American Psychiatric Association. (1952) *Diagnostic and Statistical Manual: Mental Disorders*. Washington, DC: American Psychiatric Association.

American Psychiatric Association. (1968) *Diagnostic and Statistical Manual of Mental Disorders* (2nd ed.). Washington, DC: American Psychiatric Association.

American Psychiatric Association. (1980) *Diagnostic and Statistical Manual of Mental Disorders* (3rd ed.). Washington, DC: American Psychiatric Association.

American Psychiatric Association. (2013) *Diagnostic and Statistical Manual of Mental Disorders* (5th ed.). Arlington, VA: American Psychiatric Association.

Becker, D. (1997) *Through the Looking Glass: Women and Borderline Personality Disorder*. Boulder: Westview Press.

Bourne, J. (2011) 'From Bad Character to BPD: The Medicalization of "Personality Disorder"', in Rapley, M., Moncrieff, M., and Dillon, J. (Eds.), *De-Medicalizing Misery: Psychiatry, Psychology and the Human Condition* (pp. 66–85). Houndmills, Basingstoke: Palgrave Macmillan.

Caplan, P. J. (1995) *They Say You're Crazy: How the World's Most Powerful Psychiatrists Decide Who's Normal.* Cambridge, MA: De Capo Press.

Caplan, P. J., and Cosgrove, L. (2004) 'Is This Really Necessary?', in Caplan, P. J., and Cosgrove, L. (Eds.), *Bias in Psychiatric Diagnosis* (pp. xix–xxxiii). Oxford: Jason Aronson.

Cayleff, S. E. (1988) '"Prisoners of Their Own Feebleness": Women, Nerves and Western Medicine: A Historical Overview', *Social Science & Medicine*, 26(12): 1199–1208.

Chesler, P. (2005) *Women and Madness* (rev. ed.). New York: Palgrave Macmillan.

Chrisler, J. C., and Caplan, P. (2002) 'The Strange Case of Dr. Jekyll and Ms. Hyde: How PMS Became a Cultural Phenomenon and a Psychiatric Disorder', *Annual Review of Sex Research*, 13(1): 274–306.

Decker, H. S. (2013) *The Making of DSM-III: A Diagnostic Manual's Conquest of American Psychiatry*. Oxford: Oxford University Press.

Diamond, S. (2014) 'Feminist Resistance against the Medicalization of Humanity: Integrating Knowledge about Psychiatric Oppression and Marginalized People', in Burstow, B., LeFrançois, B. A., and Diamond, S. (Eds.), *Psychiatry Disrupted: Theorizing Resistance and Crafting the (R)evolution* (pp. 194–207). Montreal & Kingston: McGill-Queen's University Press.

Ehrenreich, B., and English, D. (2005) *For Her Own Good: Two Centuries of the Experts' Advice to Women* (2nd ed.). New York: Anchor Books.

Ehrenreich, B., and English, D. (2011) *Complaints and Disorders: The Sexual Politics of Sickness* (2nd ed.). New York: The Feminist Press.

Fraad, H., Resnick, S., and Wolff, R. (1989) 'For Every Knight in Shining Armor, There's a Castle Waiting to be Cleaned: A Marxist-Feminist Analysis

of the Household', *Rethinking Marxism: A Journal of Economics, Culture & Society*, 2(4): 9–69.
Gibson, P. R. (2004) 'Histrionic Personality', in Caplan, P. J., and Cosgrove, L. (Eds.), *Bias in Psychiatric Diagnosis* (pp. 201–206). Oxford: Jason Aronson.
The Globalist. (2015) 'Women in the Workforce: A Global Perspective', *The Globalist*, http://www.theglobalist.com/women-in-the-workforce-a-global-perspective/ (retrieved on 14 April 2016).
The Globe and Mail. (2013) 'Time Spent on Domestic Labour around the World', *The Globe and Mail*, http://www.theglobeandmail.com/report-on-business/careers/career-advice/life-at-work/time-spent-on-domestic-labour--around-the-world/article12353681/?from=12300024 (retrieved on 14 April 2016).
Goldstein, J. (1982) 'The Hysteria Diagnosis and the Politics of Anticlericalism in Late Nineteenth-Century France', *Journal of Modern History*, 54(2): 209–239.
Grant Thornton. (2012) *Women in Senior Management: Still Not Enough*. Chicago: Grant Thornton International.
Haraway, D. (1978) 'Animal Sociology and a Natural Economy of the Body Politic, Part I: A Political Physiology of Dominance', *Signs: Journal of Women in Culture and Society*, 4(1): 21–36.
Hartmann, H. (1976) 'Capitalism, Patriarchy, and Job Segregation', *Signs: Journal of Women in Culture and Society*, 1(3): 137–169.
Jimenez, M. A. (1997) 'Gender and Psychiatry: Psychiatric Conceptions of Mental Disorders in Women, 1960–1994', *Affilia*, 12(2): 154–175.
Kramer, P. D. (1994) *Listening to Prozac*. London: Fourth Estate.
Kynaston, C. (1996) 'The Everyday Exploitation of Women: Housework and the Patriarchal Mode of Production', *Women's Studies International Forum*, 19(3): 221–237.
Libbon, S. E. (2007) 'Pathologizing the Female Body: Phallocentrism in Western Science', *Journal of International Women's Studies*, 8(4): 79–92.
Luhrmann, T. M. (2000) *Of Two Minds: An Anthropologist Looks at American Psychiatry*. New York: Vintage Books.
Masson, J. M. (1986) *A Dark Science: Women, Sexuality, and Psychiatry in the Nineteenth Century*. New York: Farrar, Straus and Giroux.
Masson, J. M. (1992) *The Assault on Truth: Freud's Suppression of the Seduction Theory*. New York: HarperPerennial.
Micale, M. S. (1993) 'On the "Disappearance" of Hysteria: A Study in the Clinical Deconstruction of a Diagnosis', *History of Science Society*, 84(3): 496–526.

Moncrieff, J. (2008) 'Neoliberalism and Biopsychiatry: A Marriage of Convenience', in Cohen, C. I., and Timimi, S. (Eds.), *Liberatory Psychiatry: Philosophy, Politics, and Mental Health* (pp. 235–255). Cambridge: Cambridge University Press.

Moynihan, R., and Cassels, A. (2005) *Selling Sickness: How Drug Companies are Turning Us All into Patients*. Crows Nest: Allen and Unwin.

Parker, I. (2007) *Revolution in Psychology: Alienation to Emancipation*. London: Pluto Press.

Penfold, P. S., and Walker, G. A. (1983) *Women and the Psychiatric Paradox*. Montreal: Eden Press.

Russell, D. (1995) *Women, Madness and Medicine*. Cambridge: Polity Press.

Scull, A. (2009) *Hysteria: The Disturbing History*. Oxford: Oxford University Press.

Shorter, E. (1997) *A History of Psychiatry: From the Era of the Asylum to the Age of Prozac*. New York: John Wiley & Sons.

Showalter, E. (1985) *The Female Malady: Women, Madness, and English Culture, 1830–1980*. New York: Penguin.

Smith-Rosenberg, C., and Rosenberg, C. (1973) 'The Female Animal: Medical and Biological Views of Woman and Her Role in Nineteenth-Century America', *Journal of American History*, 60(2): 332–356.

Spitzer, R. (1980) 'An In-Depth Look at DSM-III: An Interview with Robert Spitzer', *Hospital & Community Psychiatry*, 31(1): 25–32.

Stone, J., Hewett, R., Carson, A., Warlow, C., and Sharpe, M. (2008) 'The "Disappearance" of Hysteria: Historical Mystery or Illusion?', *Journal of the Royal Society of Medicine*, 101(1): 12–18.

Tseris, E., and Cohen, B. M. Z. (2016) 'Cosmetic Pharmacology', in Boslaugh, S. E. (Ed.), *The Sage Encyclopedia of Pharmacology and Society* (pp. 420–423). Thousand Oaks: Sage.

U.S. Bureau of Labor Statistics. (2014) *Women in the Labor Force: A Databook*. Washington, DC: U.S. Bureau of Labor Statistics.

Ussher, J. M. (2011) *The Madness of Women: Myth and Experience*. London: Routledge.

Veith, I. (1970) *Hysteria: The History of a Disease*. Chicago: The University of Chicago.

7

Resistance: Pathologising Dissent

The previous chapters have demonstrated that the primary function of the psy-professions is to normalise the fundamental inequalities in capitalist society as natural and common sense. The need to be constantly working on the self in the workplace, at home, and in school is reinforced through the psychiatry hegemony which has individualised and pathologised many aspects of our lived experience in neoliberal society. Predicated on the moral judgement of who is "normal" and "rational" in this society, at this historical juncture, and who is seen as abnormal and therefore in need of some sort of intervention, these professional groups are therefore fundamentally political in nature. Without a sufficient scientific base for any mental disorder (Chap. 1), the psychiatric discourse promoted at a given time is mutable to the dominant norms and values of that society. Indeed, I have argued in this book that the success that the experts of the mind have achieved within capitalism can only be fully explained through understanding the profession as an outcome of this very system; a supporting institution which furthers the needs for economic profit and, in neoliberal society, ideological control of the general population.

B.M.Z. Cohen, *Psychiatric Hegemony*,
DOI 10.1057/978-1-137-46051-6_7

The inherent political nature of the psy-disciplines has been, for the most part, successfully hidden behind their appropriation of the language and practices of scientific enquiry. This perceived objectivity and neutrality of expert knowledge on mental illness is, however, based on the liberal democratic status quo and a positioning of "normality" which is inevitably framed by the values of the free market; to disagree or rebel against such values is to risk being seen as "abnormal" and in need of "treatment" by the mental health system. As Parker (2007: 76) argues of psychologists, they "imagine that the people they study should be the same as them, that ordinary people should be neutral and impartial in judgements about the world." People who instead hold certain political opinions or, worse, are involved in collective action as part of such views are treated with suspicion and often labelled as "mentally ill" by the psy-professions. This situation is more broadly alluded to by the anti-psychiatrist, David Cooper (cited in Foucault 1988b: 191), when he states that "all madmen are political dissidents. But each delusion—or supposed delusion—may be found in political declarations."

As we shall see in this chapter, the supposed scientific discourse in psychiatry and allied disciplines has been a useful tool for pathologising collective action and political dissent within industrial society. It will be shown, for instance, that threats to the social order are reframed by the psychiatric discourse as symptoms of personal mental distress, an issue which was not lost on the civil rights leader Martin Luther King, Jnr (cited in MindFreedom 2012) in the 1950s, when he stated,

> There is a word in modern psychology which is now probably more familiar than any other words [sic] in psychology. It is the word "maladjusted" … [But] there are some things in our social system that I'm proud to be maladjusted to … I never intend to adjust myself to the viciousness of lynch mobs; I never intend to become adjusted to the evils of segregation and discrimination; I never intend to become adjusted to the tragic inequalities of the economic system which will take necessity from the masses to give luxury to the classes; I never intend to become adjusted to the insanity's of militarism, the self-defeating method of physical violence.

In every industrial society and in every epoch there are examples of psy-professions pathologising dissent and resistance to the social order. As agents of the state, these ideological institutions have defined collective struggles at various times as unlawfulness and as mental illness. As Foucault (1988b: 191, emphasis original) reminds us,

> To be dangerous *is not an offense*. To be dangerous *is not an illness*. It is not a symptom. And yet we have come, as if it is self-evident, and for over a century now, to use the notion of danger, by a perpetual movement backwards and forwards between the penal and the medical.

Indeed, the diagnostic criteria for antisocial personality disorder (APD)—the DSM-5 psychiatric label that equates closest to the mythic "sociopathic" or "psychopathic" personality types often found in psychology textbooks and popular Hollywood movies—overtly makes this connection between the violation of social norms, unlawful behaviour, and mental illness by the construction of symptoms including, "[f]ailure to conform to social norms with respect to lawful behaviors, as indicated by repeatedly performing acts that are grounds for arrest," "[d]eceitfulness, as indicated by repeated lying, use of aliases, or conning others for personal profit or pleasure," and "[c]onsistent irresponsibility, as indicated by repeated failure to sustain consistent work behavior or honor financial obligations" (American Psychiatric Association 2013: 659). The production of such psychiatric discourse holds the promise for liberal democracies and dictatorships alike of nullifying opposition and confining problematic elements on the rational basis of "medical science." In this way, psychiatric intervention has become a much more useful method of neutralisation within neoliberal society compared to the criminal justice system. This is due to the power of the mental illness label to devalue political action and collective sentiments much more effectively than the martyrdom and punishment often associated with the imprisonment of political activists.

The following discussion outlines a range of historical and contemporary examples which forward my argument for psy-professions as agents of the state and the increasing hegemonic status of the psychiatric discourse in neoliberal society. My investigation will cover psychiatry's involvement in justifying colonisation and slavery, the central role of psy-professionals in the Holocaust, and the psychiatric labelling of political dissidents as "mentally ill" in the Soviet Union. Later sections of the chapter profile more contemporary psy-practices, from the pathologisation of independence movements in Africa to their recent involvement in torturing prisoners of the "war on terror."

Biomedicine and Psychiatry's War on Race

Ongoing critiques of psychiatry's attachment to the biomedical model tend to forget one crucial factor for the institution's inability to part company with a theory which has produced so little of substance for the discipline: the legitimation of the mental health system as a true "scientific" endeavour which aligns them with other branches of medicine. As Scull (1984: 79) remarks of the introduction of mass-marketed psychopharmaceuticals in the 1950s,

> At very least, one must acknowledge that in this period [psychiatrists] were given a new treatment modality which enabled them to engage in a more passable imitation of conventional medical practice. In place of acting as glorified administrators of huge custodial warehouses, and instead of relying on crude empirical devices like shock therapy and even cruder surgical techniques like lobotomy to provide themselves with an all too transparent medical figleaf, psychiatrists in public mental hospitals could now engage in the prescription and administration of the classic symbolic accoutrement of the modern medicine man—drugs.

The successful explosion of the market in psychopharmaceuticals since the DSM-III is one of psychiatry's abiding success stories (Chap. 2). Despite the lack of any research which can conclusively identify a genetic component or a faulty neurotransmitter responsible for mental illness (Burstow 2015: 13–14), the mass marketing of mental disorders as biological disease—supported by big pharma money, a lucrative bioresearch industry and, increasingly, grassroots mental health organisations—has justified and reinforced psychiatry's expertise as the ultimate authority in the area. That this biomedically backed discourse has become hegemonic in neoliberal society is not however the result of pharmaceutical corporations themselves but rather the interests of capital more generally. While the reductionism of biological theory has been important for psychiatric legitimation within wider medicine, state and economic elites have found this discourse useful in a variety of ways, such as "scientifically" justifying colonial expansion and western imperialism, subjugating Indigenous and minority populations, oppressing social and political opposition, and in carrying out mass genocides against adults and children labelled as mentally defective or mentally ill. Key examples of these activities will be discussed in this section. It will be shown that not only has the biomedical discourse been utilised by ruling powers for such atrocities, but that psychiatry has been most enthusiastic in encouraging state support for operationalising such "science" and seeing it through, pragmatically, to its logical conclusion. This is because, like all other professional bodies, the institution of psychiatry cannot maintain their claim to an exclusive expertise and knowledge base without the support and backing of the state. This exclusivity in knowledge on mental health and illness would be seriously weakened if the main linkage to other branches of medicine—namely, the biomedical model—were to be abandoned.

In the early 1990s—at the peak of a 20-year growth in the US crime rate—the federal government announced the launch of a "violence initiative." Headed by the US Public Health Service and backed by senior psychiatrists such as Fredrick Goodwin (then chief scientist at the National Institute of Mental Health (NIMH)), this project drew on biological theories of crime which dated back to the nineteenth century Lombrosian concept of the "born criminal" (see Lombroso et al. 2006). It was proposed that a mass-screening programme of inner-city children would be undertaken across America to determine those biologically or genetically predisposed towards anti-social and violent behaviour. As a vaccine against criminality, once the "conduct-disordered" children had been identified they could then be administrated psychotropic drugs. Breggin and Breggin's (1998) detailed discussion of the violence initiative rightly demonstrates the racist ideology behind the supposed objectivity of this biomedical project; a focus on inner-city youth is blatantly a focus on minority and black communities. At the time, Goodwin allegedly made remarks at the National Advisory Mental Health Council comparing "inner-city youth to monkeys who live in a jungle, and who just want to kill each other, have sex, and reproduce" (Breggin and Breggin 1998: 4).

Psychiatry's involvement in such projects is perhaps less shocking when considering their long support for racial theories of the mind. In 1850, physician Samuel Cartwright reported in *The New Orleans Medical and Surgical Journal* his discovery of two new mental disorders affecting slaves in the Deep South: the first, drapetomania, was a disease causing slaves to run away from their owners, while the second, dysaesthesia aethiopis, resulted in the slaves becoming lazy, showing a lack of respect for the rights of property and breaking work tools (Breggin and Breggin 1998: 144–145). The prescribed cure for both disorders was "whipping, hard labor, and, in extreme cases, amputation of the toes" (Metzl 2009: 30). This psychiatric naturalisation of slavery as normal, inevitable, and even healthy for the black slave has been referred to by Burstow (2015: 37) as a blatant example of "social control medicalized." Yet as Greenberg (2013: 2–3) reminds us, for the burgeoning community of mad doctors, the discovery of such mental conditions held out the promise of contributing to contemporary society through the establishment of new "scientific" ideas in the area.

The commonalities between slavery-era diagnostic constructions and psychiatry's recent focus on inner-city youth are what Breggin and Breggin (1998: 145) describe as "the psychiatric labeling of resistive or rebellious activity in order to justify medical control." This process of enforcing the status quo through the biomedical pathologisation of the political has allowed the psychiatric profession to enhance their respectability, capital, and power in capitalist society. Though treated with suspicion by some colleagues in the north of the United States, Cartwright's ideas were widely supported by fellow physicians, local politicians, and slave owners in the south. Whereas the classifications were abruptly consigned to history by the civil war only a few years later, drapetomania, along with Kraepelin's biological theories on praecox (later relabelled as schizophrenia), were highly influential on medical researchers in the early twentieth century who contended that African Americans were "biologically unfit" for freedom (Metzl 2009: 31).

Following emancipation, incarceration rates for African Americans rose dramatically in prisons as well as asylums. This appeared to confirm the growing racialised view of black people—along with other "inferior races," including the Irish, Italians, and Chinese—within American society as less biologically evolved compared to the white population. Reflecting the opinion of many psychiatrists at the time, Metzl (2009: 31) cites the psychiatrist Arrah Evarts in 1913 as lamenting the end of slavery when she states,

> This bondage in reality was a wonderful aid to the colored man … It has been said by many observers whose words can scarce be doubted that a crazy Negro was a rare sight before emancipation. However that may be, we know he is by no means rare today.

Supporting moves towards formal segregation in America, slavery was recast by such professional opinion as a benign set of social relations between superior and inferior races in which a natural harmony had been maintained. The freed slaves were now a danger to themselves and others. As O'Malley (cited in Gambino 2008: 392) stated of black people's greater likelihood towards mental pathology in 1914,

> Before their animal appetites all barriers which society has raised in the instance of the white race go down, as though without power of frustrating … them. These appetites are gratified to such a degree that the results of these vices is a factor which has probably done more than all others to produce mental disease.

Thus, rising rates of criminality and insanity among the black population were theorised as an unsurprising and inevitable consequence of the upsetting of the "natural" racial hierarchy. All behaviours of black people on psychiatric wards were seen as further evidence of mental illness and explained using this racialised discourse. The growing rate of psychiatric incarceration for African Americans appeared to demonstrate the superiority of "civilised" white society over more "primitive" cultures. Prison rates were similarly theorised as the result of lower intelligence and the susceptibility to mental illness within these biologically "weaker" populations, with the University of Chicago sociologist Charles Henderson (cited in Gabbidon 2015: 16) arguing in 1901,

> There can be no doubt that one of the most serious factors in crime statistics is found in the conditions of the freedmen of African descent, both North and South. The causes are complex. The primary factor is racial inheritance, physical and mental inferiority, barbarism and slave ancestry and culture.

However, in an alternative reading of the situation, Du Bois (1901) pointed out that the rise in the post-emancipation prison statistics coincided with introduction of the "Black Codes," passed in many of the southern states in 1865 and 1866. These codes made it much easier for the states to incarcerate freed slaves and then return them back to the land as a prison work force.

Psychiatry's social control of the emancipated population took on the slightly more subtle biomedical approach in explaining the high levels of supposed mental illness among African Americans as a result of genetic inferiorities. The panic within white American society at the threat to the social order caused by emancipation—as well as the increased immigration of "inferior stock" from Europe—at the beginning of the twentieth century led to the growing popularity of the so-called "science" of eugenics (the study of "human improvement" by genetic means). Following the logic of biological reductionism, Galton's (1892) theory of eugenics drew on the Darwinist principles of natural selection to predict the future of the "races" (specifically, the future "quality" of the white race). For the good of humanity, argued Galton, those persons of "good quality" (by which was inferred white, middle class people of high intelligence) should be encouraged to breed only with similarly high-quality mates. In contrast, the intellectually inferior (read: the working classes in general, especially non-white groups) should be discouraged from any further reproduction. Medical scholarship was quick to support the growing arguments of the eugenics movement by producing research (e.g., through intelligence testing—see Chap. 4) which appeared to prove the superiority of the white race as a natural, evolutionary progression in the human race. Fernando (2010: 55) notes that the psy-professions supported eugenicist ideas by attributing mental illness to "inborn defects that could not be corrected." "By the middle of the twentieth century," he states, "all mental disorders were firmly set as inborn conditions."

America's eugenics policies gathered pace in the early decades of the twentieth century. By 1930, 21 states had passed laws which sanctioned the sterilisation of the "defective classes" including the mentally retarded and insane, those with epilepsy, as well as the handicapped, the criminal, and the poor (Reevy 2014: 294). The US Supreme Court was the first in history to uphold "compulsory sterilization of the insane and the 'imbecilic' [as] legal" (Burstow 2015: 48). It is estimated that over 60,000 people in the United States were sterilised as a result of such legislation (Reevy 2014: 294–295). Ironically, the increased numbers of the so-called "incurable" psychiatric patients signalled by the rising population of the asylums (Chap. 2) appeared to legitimate such Social Darwinist policies. Indeed, the "father of modern psychiatry," Emil Kraepelin, grounded the institution in the principles of scientific investigation and biomedical theory, which eventually led him to support the eugenics movement in Germany. For Kraepelin, the increased numbers of the mentally ill in the country suggested a "degeneration" of the German race (Cohen 2014a: 442). Politically useful in further ensuring exclusivity of expertise over the area of mental health and illness within society, the biomedical model has inevitably led the profession to violence, torture, and—as we shall see in the next section—genocide, all of which has been justified by the institution as in the best interests of the patient.

The Final Psychiatric Solution

Revisionist historians of medicine are keen to interpret psychiatry's enthusiastic involvement in the sterilisation and mass murder of hundreds of thousands of people labelled as "mentally ill" during the Third Reich (1933–1945) as an aberration, a perversion of correct medical practice (see, e.g., Birley 2000; Burleigh 1994; Lifton 2000). The official line is forwarded that German psychiatry was progressive, humane, and on the cutting edge of mental health care and treatment *until* the Nazis came to power in 1933. Hitler's National Socialism then manipulated the institution for its own—ultimately genocidal—ends. Thus, it is argued that a "Nazification" of German psychiatry took place, where the appropriate medical values for the care and welfare of the patient were replaced by a fascist ideology. While there were a small minority of power-hungry, racist psychiatrists who were happy to follow Hitler's orders and send mental patients to the gas chambers, such scholarship suggests that most within psychiatry remained morally opposed to and critical of the regime. Certainly, this version of events is reassuring for workers in the current mental health system, yet it is far from the truth. Belatedly, established figures in German psychiatry such as Michael von Cranach (2010: S152) have recently admitted that the psychiatric genocide was "not, as we liked to think in the first decades after the war, a small group of Nazi criminal doctors, but the majority and the elite of German psychiatrists." These seldom uttered admissions from within the profession echo the words of another psychiatrist, Frederic Wertham (cited in Breggin 1993: 135), who stated of the profession's activities during the Third Reich,

> The tragedy is that the psychiatrists did not have to have an order. They acted on their own. They were not carrying out a death sentence pronounced by someone else. They were the legislators who laid down the rules for deciding who was to die; they were the administrators who worked out the procedures, provided the patients and places, and decided the methods of killing; they pronounced a sentence of life or death in every individual case; they were the executioners who carried out or—without being coerced to do so—surrendered their patients to be killed in other institutions; they supervised and often watched the slow deaths.

"[H]ard though this may be to wrap one's head around," states Burstow (2015: 48), "psychiatrists can be reasonably theorized as architects of the Holocaust." This claim was supported by observers at the post-war Nuremberg trials, including Leo Alexander (cited in Breggin 1993: 137, emphasis added) who stated that psychiatry's operations in the 1930s could be understood as "*the entering wedge for exterminations of far greater scope* in the political program for genocide of conquered nations and the racially unwanted." Rael D. Strous (2007, emphasis original), a psychiatrist at Tel Aviv University, agrees, stating that psychiatry was

> instrumental in instituting a system of identifying, notifying, transporting, and killing hundreds of thousands of mentally ill and "racially and cognitively

> compromised" individuals in settings ranging from centralized psychiatric hospitals to prisons and death camps. Their role was *central* and *critical* to the success of Nazi policy, plans, and principles.

There was little opposition from inside the profession for the atrocities that were to follow (von Cranach 2010: S152). This is because the psychiatric profession saw these pursuits as furthering their branch of medicine, progressing biomedical ideas on the mind and the "treatment" of mental disordered patients, and—in the language of medicine under the rationale of biomedicine—in the best interests of their patients. Internationally, German psychiatry was well established, highly influential, and often considered to be at the cutting edge of new theoretical and research endeavours.

Nearly, 40 years before the Nazis came to power, in 1895, the psychologist Adolf Jost (cited in Meyer 1988: 575) published his book *The Right to Die* (Das Recht auf den Tod). In it, he argued that

> [i]n cases of incurable suffering the State can say its interest and the interest of the person concerned demand equally a quick and painless death, but it must be left to the patient to decide between life and death. In the case of mental patients this right reverts to the State, and the diagnosis of incurability is sufficient in itself to justify killing.

Jost's discussion on the state's right to kill the "incurably ill" was not out of place with the growing interest in eugenics across the psy-disciplines in western society. The book was followed in 1920 by the highly influential text, *Permission for the Extermination of Worthless Life* (Die Freigabe der Vernichtung lebensunwerten Lebens). Co-written by the lawyer Karl Binding and Alfred Hoche, a psychiatrist, the book argued for the "mercy killing" of those who were seen as an economic and social burden on the state, including "the incurably ill, the mentally ill, the feeble-minded, and deformed children" (Hassenfeld 2002: 188). Hoche gave the example of his own psychiatric institution, which he claimed was filled with people who were "incapable of human feeling and hence could have no sense of the value of life" (Hassenfeld 2002: 188). *Permission for the Extermination of Worthless Life* is widely credited with introducing the eugenic concept of the "life unworthy of living" and utilised a language that would inspire the National Socialists in due course. Burstow (2015: 48) remarks that it was no accident that psychiatry so directly inspired Nazi ideas around genetic purity and racial hygiene; "[v]ested with police powers," she says, "this was the profession whose job it had always been to protect the 'fit' from the 'unfit.' This was the profession who had taken the lead in the early theories of degeneration." Published four years later, Hitler's *Mein Kampf* (My Struggle) (cited in Breggin 1993: 137–138) was clearly influenced by the contemporary psychiatric discourse when he declared of the Nazi state that

> [i]t has to put the most modern medical means at the service of this knowledge. It has to declare unfit for propagation everybody who is visibly ill and has inherited a disease and it has to carry this out in practice ... The prevention of the procreative faculty and possibility on the part of psychiatry [sic] degenerated and mentally sick people, for only six hundred years, would not only free mankind of immeasurable misfortune, but would also contribute to a restoration that appears hardly believable today.

By the time that the Nazis were voted into office in 1933 and Hitler became German Chancellor, the German eugenics movement had been surpassed by "advances" in sterilisation policies in America (see discussion above). So often at the forefront of psychiatric scholarship and "treatments" for the mentally ill, German psychiatry felt it was falling behind the "progress" made in the United States. Towards the end of the 1933, after careful examination of the American legislation, Germany introduced the *Law for the Prevention of Offspring with Hereditary Diseases* (Das Gesetz zur Verhutung erbkranken Nachwuchses). Authored by Ernst Rudin, an internationally renowned Swiss psychiatrist and researcher on the genetics of schizophrenia (Hassenfeld 2002: 185), the Nazi's notorious sterilisation law was hailed at the time by American psychiatry as "an 'optimal example' of modern medicine" (Burstow 2015: 49). The law endowed the psychiatric apparatus in Germany with impressive new powers which were the envy of their western counterparts. The mental health system eagerly set about legally enforcing their control of the reproductive rights of the German population through enacting mandatory sterilisation orders against those labelled as mentally ill and/or physically defective. As Meyer (1988: 575–576) has outlined, those who psychiatry declared as unfit to reproduce and were therefore brought to surgical hospitals for this compulsory "treatment" included those labelled with "congenital mental deficiency, schizophrenia, cyclothymia, hereditary epilepsy, Huntington's chorea, hereditary blindness and deafness, severe malformations and severe alcoholism." Thus, a wide range of social deviants were targeted by German psychiatry for sterilisation. By 1939, 350,000 people considered as biologically unfit to reproduce had become victims of the German sterilisation law (Meyer 1988: 575).

"The next logical step," forwards Burstow (2015: 49), "was murder itself." German psychiatry's "euthanasia" programme against those they designated as mentally ill began in August 1939 with what Meyer (1988) has termed the "Action against children." This extermination programme was overseen by physicians and psychiatrists, and rationalised in the name of biomedicine under the guise of acting in the best interests of the patient. Under the organisation of the Federal Board for the Scientific Registration of Hereditary or Other Severe Congenital Diseases, German children designated by medical staff as "disabled" or "mentally abnormal" were sent to so-called Specialised Children's Departments—effectively, child extermination centres (Seeman 2005: 222). Information on these children was reviewed by a panel of three medical experts in Berlin—two paediatricians and the psychiatrist Hans Heinze (Breggin and Breggin 1998: 126). No personal examination was made of the child and often no case histories were available (Meyer 1988: 576). If a decision for "treatment" was met by the panel, the child would be killed by what has been described by Breggin and Breggin (1998: 126–127) as a "tortuous method" whereby doctors and nurses utilised "a combination of gradual poisoning with toxic drugs and slow starvation." Unlike other genocides committed during the Third Reich, the children's Action continued right up until the end of the war, with the scope of those children coming under the auspices of the programme extending from three to 17 years old (Meyer 1988: 576). In this way, a total of up to 6000 children were murdered (Burleigh 1994: 223). The medical staff involved in this genocide against children justified their actions as in the patient's best interest; it was ultimately the correct goal of medicine to "release unfortunate creatures from their suffering"

(Burleigh 1994: 223). At the end of the war, Werner Catel (the paediatrician who headed the programme) was more forthright in his belief that the medical project had simply performed a public service in murdering what he still referred to at his trial as "monsters." "[C]omplete morons," he argued, "when considered even from a religious point of view, are not human beings as they have no personality. To exterminate them is neither murder nor killing" (cited in Meyer 1988: 576).

The psychiatric system of bureaucratised genocide installed with the Action against children programme formed the operational basis for the much larger "mercy killings" of the adult "insane" and "disabled" populations instigated with the notorious Action T4 (named after the central office of operations, at No. 4 Tiergartenstrasse in Berlin). This was a programme of systematic mass murder that was later utilised to carry out the Holocaust against the Jews and other "undesirable groups" (including the Roma population, communists, and homosexuals). Action T4 may have had Nazi support, but Hitler firmly left the process of evaluating those to be "euthanised"—and the means by which it would happen—in psychiatry's hands. In 1939, he charged the Würzburg professor of psychiatry, Werner Heyde, with setting up a team of 30 psychiatric experts—many of whom were senior university professors (Hassenfeld 2002: 188)—to give "careful consideration" of each patient's medical condition to determine who would "be accorded a mercy death" (cited in Meyer 1988: 577). Significantly, this "Euthanasia Decree" from the Chancellor was not a law; as Strous (2007, emphases added) states, "[p]sychiatrists were … *never ordered* to facilitate the process or carry out the murder of [the] mentally ill," however, "they were *empowered* to do so." It was a decree that further heightened psychiatry's power within the state, and one which the institution took to with a genocidal verve.

Action T4 required that all psychiatric hospitals complete a questionnaire on each individual patient. Including information on diagnosis, length of stay, and the extent of disability, the resulting surveys for each patient were assessed by three from the team of 30 experts. No personal examination of the inmate was made by the psychiatrists. The consultants' only purpose was to make a decision from the questionnaire as to whether the patient should be put to death or allowed to live (Hassenfeld 2002: 187). Records show that within a two week period in 1939, one expert made decisions on 2100 patients (Meyer 1988: 577). By 1941, psychiatric staff had ordered and carried out the mass murder of up to 100,000 people in Germany (Breggin 1993: 134), with those considered long-term inmates, "criminally insane," of "unpure blood," or unable to work particularly likely to receive a death sentence (Meyer 1988: 577).

The extermination of so many psychiatric inmates would not have been possible without Action T4's establishment of six killing centres—known as "euthanasia institutions"—across Germany, at Brandenburg, Grafeneck, Hartheim, Sonnenstein, Bernburg, and Hadamar (Strous 2006: 27). Significantly, these were the first institutions to install gas chambers disguised as communal showers, as well as crematoriums to dispose of the large number of bodies. Those condemned to death by psychiatry were transferred in their hundreds from hospitals to the centres by so-called "grey buses." "On arrival to the killing institutions," recounts von Cranach (2010: S153-S154), "the patients were undressed and led to the gas chamber. A team of doctors and nurses observed the dying process of the patients." Over time, these institutions of mass murder became increasingly "efficient" in their organisational processes of killing, with Strous (2006: 27) noting of the Hadamar institution (near Wiesbaden) that it had approximately 100 staff working there in 1941—weighing, photographing, and supervising each patient into the gas chamber and, later, removing "various organs for medical research," the bodies then being "buried in mass graves located on the hospital grounds." As with the Action against children, a medical registry was set up at these institutions to produce false death certificates and send letters of condolence to the relatives. "The latter," notes Meyer (1988: 577), "were told that the body had already been cremated by order of the police because of the risk of epidemics."

Action T4 was formally ended in August 1941. This happened for two specific reasons according to von Cranach (2010: S154): "increasing public criticism on the one side and the transfer of this killing technology [i.e. the apparatus of the euthanasia centres] to the newly built concentration camps in Poland on the other." Breggin (1993: 135) correctly states that psychiatry had successfully pioneered processes of mass killing that could now be used to see through Hitler's "Final Solution," namely "medical experts to justify the killings as medical procedures, gas chambers disguised as showers, and the mass cremation of bodies to avoid legal entanglements over corpses." Alongside the physical apparatus from the institutions, some of the most senior and experienced psychiatric staff from the euthanasia centres were transferred to the large concentration camps in the East. These physicians oversaw the initial organisation and implementation of the gas chambers in advisory roles, though in the case of the psychiatrist Irmfried Eberl, he became the first commandant of the Treblinka death camp (Breggin 1993: 136). Under the direction of Action T4's Werner Heyde, psychiatrists also carried out the first systematic murder of concentration camp inmates in a euthanasia centre, almost as a genocidal "practice run" for the Holocaust to follow. Using diagnostic criteria and the euthanasia questionnaire to now select (overtly) "racial" and "political" types for extermination, it is estimated that 10,000 prisoners were murdered by Heyde's psychiatric team (Breggin 1993: 136). Further, the original euthanasia programme was introduced to the concentration camps under the code name "Aktion 14f13" to "rid the camps of sick prisoners" (Seeman 2005: 222); as many as a 100,000 inmates considered as either "disabled" or "mentally ill" by the camp physicians were sent to the gas chambers as a result of this programme.

Action T4 was also halted by a growing unease from the German public—as well as from the Nazi hierarchy—as to the ruthlessness with which psychiatry had carried out the murders of over 70,000 of their own "sick" citizens (most of whom were still considered Aryan, even if their genetic "strength" could be biomedically questioned by their supposed mental illness). Hitler ordered an end to the killing and a cessation of Action T4; it was not an issue worth perusing at the time, when the facilities created by psychiatry could be better utilised against "foreign" elements in the East. However, far from the cancellation of Action T4 signalling the end of mass murder within the mental health system, "psychiatrists essentially doubled their effort" (Burstow 2015: 50) with a period described in Nazi documents of the time as "wild euthanasia" (Seeman 2005: 222). Psychiatry did not need to be handed state decrees to begin a programme of extermination against those labelled as "mental ill," and they certainly did not need one to continue the killing. Instead, belief in biomedical progress meant that the institution continued to perform what they believed was a justifiable medical service for the greater good of the nation. Seeman (2005: 222) recounts that "[f]rom 1941 onward, patients who suffered from mental illness were killed by neglect and starvation and, when this method proved too slow, by lethal injection." With the selection criteria of the T4 euthanasia questionnaires no longer a restriction on this "medical practice," psychiatry reverted to type, seeking to rid Germany of any deviant or socially problematic group they could identify and bring under their jurisdiction. This included homosexuals, criminals, residents of reform schools, the elderly, the poor, the hard to manage, and slave labourers who were physically ill (Seeman 2005: 222). Conservative estimates suggest that at least 70,000 were murdered during the "wild euthanasia" phase of the psychiatric genocide (Breggin 1993: 134). It has been documented that, by the end of the war, some of the larger psychiatric institutions in Germany were completely empty, every inmate having been executed by the mental health staff (Breggin 1993: 135).

As the allied forces closed in on Germany in 1945, the death camps were shut down or abandoned by the Nazis. The psychiatric killings, however, continued. With unabated enthusiasm, the mass murders progressed right up until end of the war, and are documented as having continued in some institutions even after this point (Breggin 1993: 134). The testimony of a young officer, Robert Abrams, is poignant in this regard: three weeks into allied occupation, Abrams was alerted by a German physician to rumours of a psychiatric facility in the village of Kaufbeuren (near Munich) where psychiatrists killed their patients. On arrival, he found the medical staff carrying out the murders as normal, something that was only halted under the threat of being shot (Burstow 2015: 50). Abrams stated of the hospital staff who had witnessed and taken part in the atrocities: "[t]he nurses belonged to religious orders," while "a psychiatrist who led him through the hospital showed no remorse. He was not a Nazi party member, and believed that he had acted in the name of medicine" (Breggin 1993: 134).

Very soon after the war, states von Cranach (2010: S154), "knowledge about the killing of the patients was repressed. Manuscripts on the topic found no publishers, or their distribution was hampered." This situation generally remains in psychiatry today with Strous (2007) noting that "[l]ittle has been published on the subject [of the killings] in mainstream psychiatry journals and even less is part of the formal education process for medical students and psychiatry residents." Significantly, Edward Shorter's

A History of Psychiatry (1997)—one of the most popular official texts on the profession's history—completely ignores the period (as does Lieberman's perhaps ironically titled recent history, *Shrinks: the Untold Story of Psychiatry* (2015)). Despite the estimated 250,000–300,000 patients murdered across Europe at the hands of the mental health system (Breggin 1993: 135), only one physician who worked in the euthanasia programme was ever brought to justice (Breggin and Breggin 1998: 127). Many continued to work as mental health professionals under allied or Russian occupation following the war. Some even went on to receive high accolades. Elizabeth Hecker, for example, a child and adolescent psychiatrist in the Third Reich who regularly reported children with low intelligence for transfer to the local "special department" for execution, was made an honorary member of the German Association of Child and Adolescent Psychiatry in 1979, for her "postwar commitment to the cause" (Seeman 2005: 223).

The psychiatric genocide in Germany was no aberration of medicine but rather a logical consequence of the application of biomedical reductionism to social deviance. While the systematic mass murder of psychiatric inmates was unique within the profession's history, all other biomedical "treatments" of the Third Reich's mental health system were being utilised in other countries. Indeed, Breggin (1993: 140) notes that the mass sterilisations in Germany could not subsequently be classified as a war crime because "they were international in scope, representative of psychiatric activities throughout the western world." The use of biological theory by the profession to label social deviants as inherently "abnormal," "defective," or "mental ill" has been conducive to both authoritarian and liberal democratic societies alike. While the rise of National Socialism was useful to the profession in allowing them to "advance" their areas of "expertise" and sites of jurisdictional power, it was psychiatry itself that advanced the argument that minority groups posed a threat to the future of society and promoted the racist ideology of eugenics. What may seem peculiar—not to mention unethical, inhumane, and immoral—from the outside is business as usual for institutions of social control such as psychiatry. The murderous practices of German psychiatry in the Third Reich were soon written off by official historians of medicine as a "political abuse of psychiatry" (see, e.g., Birley 2000), and the institution resumed its practices of physical and ideological oppression of state opposition.

Colonial Resistance and Psychiatry's "Civilising" Principle

Despite the atrocities committed by the mental health system in the Third Reich, psy-professions continued to flourish post-war and expand into new territories. Counter-intuitively, psychiatry had proved its worth as an effective institution of social control within industrial societies—medicalising protest as symptoms of mental illness was a much more effective way of devaluing and pacifying oppositional movements, as opposed to the direct and more overt oppression at the hands of the judicial system. For example, in the Soviet Union, psychiatrists utilised the diagnosis of "sluggish schizophrenia"—theorised by psychiatrists as involving symptoms such as "philosophical intoxication" and "delusions of reformism" (Park et al. 2014: 365)—to label political dissidents as mentally ill, a situation which only intensified in the decades following the death of Stalin in 1953 (Healey 2014: 78–80; Keukens and van Voren 2007: S4). In fact, the belief in this label by Soviet psychiatry was so strong that when the General Secretary of the Communist Party, Mikhail Gorbachev, began to speak the language of reform in the mid-1980s, some worried that he was showing all the signs of having this mental illness (van Voren 2002: 132–133). From the Cultural Revolution of the 1960s onwards, forensic psychiatry in China has also increased its labelling of political resistance as symptoms of mental illness; open and active dissent against the government is understood by the mental health system as delusions of persecution, paranoia, and delusions of grandeur, for which the patient is most readily diagnosed with schizophrenia (Munro 2002: 99–100). Significantly, Munro (2002: 100) notes that many such cases in China appeared in 1978 and 1989, two years which witnessed an upsurge in protest and civil disobedience in the country (the former, the Democracy Wall movement, and the latter, the Tiananmen Square pro-democracy demonstrations). Elsewhere, systematic policing of political resistance by the psychiatric system has also been recently reported in Romania and Cuba (Keukens and van Voren 2007: S4).

All of the above cases have been highlighted by western psychiatrists themselves as examples of the continuing misuse of the mental health system in state socialist societies. Ironically, these commentators are usually falling over themselves to argue that politically oppressed groups within such "undemocratic" mental health systems are categorically sane (see, e.g., Bonnie 2002; Healey 2014; van Voren 2010), despite counter-commentaries from local psychiatric staff declaring that they are appropriately assessing potential patients to the same standards as their western colleagues without any political involvement (see, e.g., Lee and Kleinman 2002; Stone 2002). The insinuation from western psychiatry is that, based on liberal democratic principles, their own work is free from the political ideology and oppressive practices which plague their colleagues elsewhere. As Hickling (2002: 112) has outlined, however, this critique only demonstrates further the hegemonic role such professionals play in western society. "The Western ideologues," he explains,

> enlist professional custodians of their ideology to attack and discredit all the legal and definitional principles of the opposing ideology. The Western ideologues see no contradiction in their own abuse of individual freedoms within the disciplines of criminology and psychiatry if these acts of political misuse and abuse are perpetrated against individuals or racial groups who are outside their own preferred purview.

Yet mental health systems across the globe have a distinct commonality in the labelling, incarcerating, and "treating" of groups considered deviant and, thus, a potential threat to society. As a supporting institution of capitalism, western psychiatry has sought to neutralise the inevitable contradictions created by capital (e.g., the increasingly disparities in income and wealth) through pathologising political threats to the social order as symptoms of individual mental disorder. This section will discuss a number of key examples of this process by focusing on psychiatry's response to Indigenous struggles for independence from western imperialism, as well as the US civil rights movement of the 1960s and 1970s.

As the psy-professionals' support of Social Darwinism and eugenics had aided the Holocaust, so these ideas also helped rationalise colonial expansion of the western powers across Africa and Asia in the nineteenth and twentieth centuries. The violent theft of land, destruction of local cultures, and genocide of Indigenous peoples through famine, war, and systematic murder were all justified as part of the "white man's burden" to bring "civilisation" to "primitive" societies. As biological theory had been used to justify the enslavement and incarceration of black and minority groups in the west, it was similarly used by the psy-professions on colonised populations to characterise them as inherently inferior.

Western psychiatry expanded its jurisdiction into new territories through aiding western imperialism as an institution of social control. In enforcing the norms and values of Empire as the only correct and true principles for governance, colonial psychiatry served to normalise colonial rule while pathologising Indigenous resistance. Rather than acknowledging political activism and armed struggle as normal and necessary responses to the imposition of foreign rule, colonial psychiatry utilised the language of medical science to label and silence opposition. As Roman et al. (2009: 19) have stated of the imposition of colonial authority on the First Nations people of Canada, colonial psychiatry was "used to advance colonial nation-building and the very definition of civil society—its boundaries between the so-called 'fit' and 'unfit' citizens, indeed the very uses of psychiatric practices intertwined with legal practices in a fledgling settler-state." Thus, the chief imperative of the introduction of western mental health services to the colonies was to naturalise the ongoing oppression of local populations. This was achieved through a psychologised language which depoliticised the violence and trauma of colonisation; as Vaughan (2007: 2) remarks, "colonial psychiatrists offered an analysis of social evolution, and a scientific language in which to discuss a range of vexing behavioural traits amongst colonized peoples, from excessive docility to outright rebellion."

The cultural hegemony of the Empire was reinforced through the biological theories of western mental health workers; in this way, Keller (2007: 4) argues that "[p]sychiatry brought a new degree of sophistication to colonial racism." A common thread which ran through such psychological theory was that "there was something abnormal about the 'normal' native mind" (Vaughan 2007: 11). For example, the Malay in the Dutch-occupied East Indies were conceptualised as "over emotional," the Indigenous populations of British-occupied East Africa as being sent mad by "detribalization" (Vaughan 2007: 11), and North African Muslims of French-occupied Algeria as suffering from a "persecution complex" (Cohen 2014b: 320). Given the role of psychiatry in the colonies, it is unsurprising that their systematic stereotyping and labelling of the Indigenous "other" intensified as the struggles for independence grew in 1950s and 1960s. The outbreak of guerrilla war and acts of political violence against western powers was theorised by the profession as an alarming example of the inherent immaturity and instability of the native mind which could lead to psychotic episodes of violence if left untreated. These attempts by western mental health experts to pacify resistance to colonial authority was discussed in detail by the famous psychiatrist and social theorist Frantz Fanon (1965: 200), who wrote at the time of the Algerian War of Independence (1954–1962),

> We cannot be held responsible that in this war psychiatric phenomena entailing disorders affecting behaviour and thought have taken on importance where those who carry out the "pacification" are concerned, or that these same disorders are notable among the "pacified" population. The truth is that colonialism in its essence was already taking on the aspect of a fertile purveyor for psychiatric hospitals. We have since 1954 in various scientific works drawn the attention of both French and international psychiatrists to the difficulties that arise when seeking to "cure" a native properly, that is to say, when seeking to make him thoroughly a part of a social background of the colonial type.

As the writings of Fanon and Gandhi inspired independence movements in Africa and Asia, so they gave hope to struggles against white rule in other parts of the world including Apartheid South Africa and the similarly segregated United States. As black, Indigenous, and minority protest and collective action for equal rights grew across western societies in the 1960s and 1970s, psy-professionals intensified their focus on these movements as "dangerous" in a similar way to that of their colonial colleagues. Racial ideology was again utilised to theorise the rising tide of political action as symptoms of pathology. For example, previously conceptualised as a passive and simpler "race" of people by biomedical psychiatry in America, the view of Africa Americans radically transformed in the 1960s (Metzl 2009).

Through research on cultural documents and clinical evidence, Metzl notes how the use of the schizophrenia diagnosis changed from describing "sensitive," white, middle class patients between the 1920s and the

1950s, to a signifier for a growing population of "violent" young black men. As Metzl (2009: xiii) reiterates,

> American assumptions about race, gender, and temperament of schizophrenia changed beginning in the 1960s. Many leading medical and popular sources suddenly described schizophrenia as an illness manifested not by docility, but by rage. Growing numbers of research articles from leading psychiatric journals asserted that schizophrenia was a condition that also afflicted "Negro men," and that black forms of illness were marked by volatility and aggression. In the worst cases, psychiatric authors conflated the schizophrenic symptoms of African American patients with the perceived schizophrenia of civil rights protests, particularly those organized by Black Power, Black Panthers, Nation of Islam, or other activist groups.

Adverts for anti-psychotics during the period played on the popular image of the out-of-control black man. One advert reproduced by Metzl (2009: xiv) shows a black man with a clenched fist: "[a]ssaultive and belligerent?," asks the headline, "[c]ooperation often begins with [the anti-psychotic drug] HALDOL." A similar process of medicalising protest and political resistance has been documented in my own research on the Māori "cultural renaissance" of the 1960s and 1970s (see Cohen 2014b). According to psychiatric authorities and government statistics, until the 1950s, Māori—the Indigenous people of Aotearoa, New Zealand—were mentally healthier than settler populations. This situation drastically changed in the following decades, with a significant rise in psychiatric incarceration (especially for those aged between 20 and 30 years old) and rates of psychoses for Māori. By 1973, the psychologist Richard Kelly was suggesting that the typical image of the Māori held by the white colonisers was in need of revision. The aggressive and deluded personality traits which accompanied a psychosis diagnosis meant that the evidence now stood "in marked contrast to the stereotype commonly held by the [white] European of a simple, good natured, relaxed and often lazy people" (Kelly 1973: 729).

This pervading view of the Indigenous people as increasingly psychotic coincided with what is known locally as the Māori cultural renaissance. Influenced by the civil rights movement in the United States as well as countercultural philosophies and global struggles against colonial power, Māori organisations emerged in the 1960s as a direct challenge to the authority of the British Crown. Political protests and forms of direct action around the country—including land rights marches, occupations and protests at public and sporting events, and other acts of civil disobedience—sought to highlight the systematic theft of Māori land and cultural genocide which had taken place since the imposition of white rule in 1840. Walker (1990: 220) rightly conceptualises the formation of a growing political consciousness among the Indigenous people—particularly the young people—during the 1960s and 1970s as a direct challenge to the hegemony of colonial authority. White society was frightened by what appeared to be an increasingly angry and aggressive Māori population, and psychiatry's latent colonial function in the British colony was enacted through the labelling and incarcerating of increasing numbers of the Indigenous population.

The findings of my research support Metzl's theorising on the US civil rights movement as well as the critical scholarship on colonial psychiatry; as a supporting institution of white rule, the mental health system has demonstrated its ability across the globe to reframe legitimate protest and struggle against an oppressive social order as symptoms of major mental illness. Respected psychiatrist and social critic Suman Fernando (2010: 61–73) has drawn attention to the continuation of these systematic practices within the western mental health system as examples of institutionalised racism (see also Kutchins and Kirk 1997: 200–237). Specifically, he highlights British psychiatry's construction and use of the "cannabis psychosis" classification in the 1980s (see full discussion in McGovern and Cope 1987)—a diagnosis which pathologised the growing anger of a disenfranchised young, black population in Margaret Thatcher's Britain as due to smoking marijuana. "On both sides of the Atlantic," states Fernando (2010: 23), "vicious circles have developed with myths about degeneracy of blacks becoming 'facts' of diagnosed psychoses through the collaboration of psychiatry." A situation which, as we have seen in this discussion, has a long tradition in psychiatry, from slavery, eugenics, and the Holocaust to colonial resistance, the civil rights movement, and the "violence initiative."

The Culture of Fear and the War without End

As previous sections of this chapter have demonstrated, the institution of psychiatry and its supporting professions have been responsible for the moral policing of political protest and collective action which threatens the dominant social order. The inherent contradictions of capitalism bring forth continuous points of collective resistance, some recent examples being the World Trade Organisation/Anti-Globalisation protests, the Stop the War coalition, and the global Occupy movement. As a supporting institution of capital the role of the mental health system is to delegitimise such political action as signs of irrationality, dangerousness, and mental pathology rather than a rational and logical consequence of widening social and economic disparities within western society.

Following the 9/11 attacks, the US government's "war on terror"—in which millions of people in the Middle East and Afghanistan have been killed, the region has become increasingly unstable and prone to civil war, and has eventuated in a humanitarian epidemic of outward migration across Europe—constructed a popular (if old fashioned) western rhetoric of good versus evil in which, according to President George W. Bush, you were either "with us, or against us" (cited in Hickling 2002: 118). Appreciators of George Orwell were quick to point out the similarities between Bush's polemic and the "war without end" from his classic novel *1984*. Days after the twin tower attacks, at a massive peace march in Berlin, the American Ambassador to Germany used sympathy for the American dead to call for our support for a war which could last long into the foreseeable future against elements which were, to a large extent, unknown. The seemingly endless war that the Ambassador foretold that day at the Brandenburg Gate and the heightened "culture of fear" against a "terrorist" other has been useful in facilitating the expansion of the dubious knowledge base and practices of mental health "experts" in the twenty-first century. In this discussion I will briefly outline three ways in which this has happened: first, through medicalising criminal and political violence, thereby delegitimising internal and external threats to capital; second, through the expansion of diagnostic practice and the political economy of mental health on the basis of the increased fear and anxiety of violent attacks on western populations; and thirdly, in directly facilitating the western allies' programme of torture and terrorism against civilian populations under the guise of humane doctoring practices.

Geopolitical events of the past 15 years have had their effects on the psychiatric discourse. Specifically, there has been an increased focus on the figure of the dangerous agitator and the violent "terrorist." For example, Table 7.1 shows results from my textual analysis of protest-related words and phrases in each edition of the DSM. Notable is the APA's tripling in the use of the "violent" and "violence" phrasings in categories of mental illness between the DSM-IV-TR in 2000 and the DSM-5 in 2013. This is used to pathologise both the victims of violence—through classifications such as PTSD or BPD (Tseris 2013)—as well as those who perpetuate it, individualising acts of political violence as those of sick individuals rather than the rational behaviour of oppressed or marginalised groups. As Parker (2007: 86) has stated of the depoliticising discourse in psychology,

> [T]he awful choices that groups make are abstracted from the contradictory conditions in which they are forced to act, and the "psychological" bit of the explanation makes it seem like the bad choice must be based on faulty reasoning or mental pathology.

The attempt to delegitimise those involved in acts of political violence is also evidenced by the introduction of a new mental illness in the DSM-5—other specified dissociative disorder (OSDD). This mental

Table 7.1 Number of protest-related words/phrases in the DSM, 1952–2013[a]

Word/phrase	DSM-I (1952)	DSM-II (1968)	DSM-III (1980)	DSM-III-R (1987)	DSM-IV (1994)	DSM-IV-TR (2000)	DSM-5 (2013)
Delusions of persecution/ paranoia	10	7	31	19	5	3	14
Violent/ce	1	4	38	40	41	43	148
Self-control	0	0	0	1	1	1	10
Police/ing	0	0	4	4	6	5	7
Socio/politics/al	0	0	6	7	8	9	13
Terror/ist/ism	0	0	1	1	2	2	9
Total count	11	11	80	72	63	63	201

[a]See Appendix A for methodology

pathology suggests that rational people would not voluntarily choose to undertake such actions; instead, the APA state that those suffering from OSDD have experienced an "identity disturbance due to prolonged and intense coercive persuasion" (American Psychiatric Association 2013: 306). Critical questioning or consciousness of oppressive conditions under capitalism can only be understood by psychiatry as symptoms of a mental disorder, the DSM-5 (American Psychiatric Association 2013: 306) adding of those with OSDD that "[i]ndividuals who have been subjected to intense coercive persuasion (e.g., brainwashing, thought reform, indoctrination while captive, torture, long-term political imprisonment, recruitment by sects/cults or by terror organizations) may present with prolonged changes in, or conscious questioning of, their identity."

It is also of note in Table 7.1 that the APA is again increasing its use of "delusions of persecution" and "paranoia" within diagnostic categories. These are phrases which we have previously seen used by colonial psychiatry—as well as in China—against political dissidents and protest movements (see above discussion). Schizophrenia, a diagnosis which Szasz (1988) describes as psychiatry's "sacred symbol," continues to be a label often utilised to describe troublesome, dangerous, and problematic elements for capital. However, the all-purpose category to define those who defy the moral order and break the law remains APD—a label which featured in the first DSM in 1952 but has taken on increasing significance in the new millennium (McCallum 2001). The label was introduced in the DSM-I to pathologise and irrationalise criminal behaviour, yet with the expansion of the neoliberal doctrine and the resulting protests and actions against financial disparities, the symptoms and features of APD have expanded and the language used in the diagnosis has become increasingly personal and disdainful. For example, under the features supporting a diagnosis of APD, the DSM-5 states (American Psychiatric Association 2013: 660) that such individuals

> may have an inflated and arrogant self-appraisal (e.g., feel that ordinary work is beneath them or lack a realistic concern about their current problems or their future) and may be excessively opinionated, self-assured, or cocky. They may display a glib, superficial charm and can be quite voluble

> and verbally facile (e.g., using technical terms or jargon that might impress someone who is unfamiliar with the topic).

Essentially, those labelled with APD are dangerous individuals who cannot be trusted, will often break the law, are likely be incarcerated, and are doomed by the APA to a shorter life than the rest of us. To quote the DSM-5 (American Psychiatric Association 2013: 661) again, those with APD

> may receive dishonorable discharges from the armed services, may fail to be self-supporting, may become impoverished or even homeless, or may spend many years in penal institutions. Individuals with antisocial personality disorder are more likely than people in the general population to die prematurely by violent means (e.g., suicide, accidents, homicides).

APD is the perfect catch-all label with which to devalue and pathologise the behaviour of anyone who breaks legal or moral codes in society, particularly those who demonstrate violent conduct (including on picket lines, marches, at occupations, and during other acts of civil disobedience).

The irony of psy-professions' focus on political violence as symptoms of pathology is the denial of their own involvement in inflicting systematic institutional violence on others. The discussion in this chapter has already alerted the reader to the inherent tendencies of the mental health experts to carry out acts of torture and genocide against groups of social deviants who threaten the social order. Described by Nathaniel Raymond of Physicians for Human Rights as "arguably the single greatest medical-ethics scandal in American history" (cited in Mayer 2009), a contemporary case in point is the American Psychological Association's involvement in the torture of detainees at US military prisons at Abu Ghraib and Guantanamo Bay (also the topic of the 2011 documentary film, *Doctors of the Dark Side*). Echoing psychiatry's involvement in the Holocaust, this is another example of the role of the mental health system in legitimating the violent oppression of political opposition in exchange for increased professional power.

The events of 9/11 offered a prime opportunity for the American Psychological Association to extend their areas of jurisdiction by making themselves indispensable to the "war on terror." In Philip Zimbardo, the Association had a president who understood the importance of the psychological sciences making their skills directly available to state agencies. Mirroring the rhetoric of President Bush, Zimbardo argued at the time that psychologists should put aside their differences in the face of the "cults of hatred" currently aligned against the United States (cited in Parker 2007: 89). The attack on the twin towers, he contended, "provided psychology with an unprecedented obligation and opportunity to collectively serve society" (Zimbardo 2002: 433), one which called for "a new kind of psychological warfare" (Zimbardo 2002: 432). Under his presidency, Zimbardo promised that much closer cooperation with leaders and policymakers would be possible if psychology could prove their usefulness to the state. "I sincerely believe," he wrote in 2002, "that as psychology focuses on its most recent societal obligations, the nation's highest level of elected officials will become more responsive to psychologists' unique needs and talents" (Zimbardo 2002: 433).

Psychology's unique talents have since become public knowledge, thanks to the investigative reporting of Katherine Eban for *Vanity Fair* and James Risen of the *New York Times*. As confirmed in the recent independent review on ethics, national security and torture for the American Psychological Association (Hoffman et al. 2015), both reporters uncovered not only the Association's sanctioning of psychologists' and behavioural scientists' involvement in the Bush government's "enhanced interrogation techniques" (i.e., forms of torture such as water boarding, sleep deprivation, and forced nakedness) at Abu Ghraib and Guantanamo Bay, but also the organisation's systematic coordination of policy changes on "ethics" which knowingly make it easier for their members to participate in such practices without the threat of professional or legal reprisals. As outlined in Risen's book *Pay Any Price: Greed, Power, and Endless War* (2014), this was not the result of a small number of strategically placed individuals who somehow corrupted the American Psychological Association and tarnished their good name, but instead involved the profession as a whole. While many psychologists were not directly involved in the US government's torture practices and may even have been morally opposed to them, they were all benefiting economically and professionally from the closer association with state power which Zimbardo had promised them. No one within the profession suggested that their involvement in torture practices was out of keeping with psychology's purpose and high ethical standards of care.

No strangers to carrying out "interrogation research" for the military and other state authorities, the American Psychological Association was well aware that torture was not an effective way of eliciting accurate information from prisoners. Yet they remained silent on this issue. "Worse," states Risen (2014: 178), "they participated, and quietly changed their profession's ethics code to allow torture to continue. In return the psychologists were showered with government money and benefits." In 2005, the response of psychologists to reports of their complicity in the torture programmes was the American Psychological Association's Presidential Task Force on Psychological Ethics and National Security (PENS). The involvement of psychologists in the torture of inmates at US facilities, concluded PENS, was "appropriate and ethical … in order to ensure that [the interrogations] remained safe, legal, ethical, and effective" (Risen 2014: 197). If some wondered that this position sounded very much like the double-speak of the Bush government to justify their use of violence, it has since been confirmed by Risen (2014: 197–200) that the first drafts of the American Psychological Association's 2005 ethics code were indeed produced in close cooperation with the Central Intelligence Agency (CIA) and the Pentagon (in fact, early negotiations on the issue had taken place between these parties long before PENS was even formed). In 2007, the Association again reinforced their support for the methods of torture by rejecting a proposal which would have banned psychologists from taking part in interrogations "in which detainees are deprived of adequate protection of their human rights" (cited in Welch 2010: 133). As Risen (2014: 192) has noted, few within the American Psychological Association had qualms "about getting involved with institutions [such as the CIA and the Pentagon] that were using pseudo behavioral science to brutalize prisoners," and in fact the revision of their ethics policies allowed the psychologists involved in torture to prioritise a "governing legal authority" if their practices ever conflicted with the Association's own code of ethics (Risen 2014: 194–195). This was a change that echoed the Nuremburg defence for American psychology—"following lawful orders was an acceptable reason to violate professional ethics" (Risen 2014: 195).

The involvement of the psy-professions in the "war on terror" has been crucial to western governments in legitimating violence against war combatants and civil populations as seemingly legal, if not humane. As Welch (2010: 133) has argued of the American Psychological Association's recent involvement in practices of torture,

> With a veneer of science, advocates of "enhanced" interrogation claim that those who administer such techniques are "experts" and "professionals" committed to national security. Therefore, the entire interrogation program may be viewed by some observers—and participants—as humane since licensed psychologists supervise it.

Similarly, involvement with the highest levels of office increases psy-professional power and spheres of influence. Only a few American psychologists were given multi-million dollar contracts from the government to facilitate the torture programme, more benefited from a boost in their research funding, publications, and paid appearances at security service seminars on interrogation techniques. However, the heightened status and perceived usefulness to state powers of such psychological practices has benefited mental health institutions as a whole. In the case of the American Psychological Association, Risen (2014: 196–197) saliently places them in the wider context of the struggle with the psychiatric profession for dominance of the mental health field; making themselves useful to state powers holds out the promise of an extension of prescription rights to American psychologists, something that is currently restricted to psychologists who work in military hospitals. As Zimbardo himself has admitted, above all else what the profession was hoping to achieve in the new millennium was "prescription privileges" (cited in Risen 2014: 197).

Risen's (2014) book alerts us to the amount of money and power that has been accumulated by professional bodies and institutions that have promoted a post-9/11 "culture of fear." As we have seen in this section, psy-professionals are no exception; on the contrary, they have played a central role in supporting the ideological "war on terror" while pathologising civil disobedience and political protest. The contemporary priorities of the experts on the mind are not simple errors in judgement.

Instead, reiterates Parker (2007: 91), they "follow the political logic of the cultural ideological context in which they work." It is a hegemonic discourse that justifies the maintenance and expansion of western capital by continuing to racialise and depoliticise popular dissent, whether vocalised at the national or international level. Thus, summates Parker (2007: 90), "the civil wars in Iraq and Afghanistan boil down to a 'clash of civilizations' rather than a history of subjugation and then invasion by imperialist powers." In this way, the mental illness discourse in neoliberal society can be understood as the continuation of a racist ideology which has benefited the psychiatric profession since the beginning of industrial society.

Summary

This chapter has explored some of the most blatant ways in which the western system of mental health has sought to medicalise dissent. As a conservative and morally controlling force within capitalist society, I have discussed how the psy-professions have increased their professional capital and power through promoting a psychiatric discourse which serves to incarcerate, torture, and murder political opposition and deviant groups under the rhetoric of "medical progress" and "acting in the best interests of the patient." Reflecting the argument of this book, psychiatrist Frederick Hickling (2002: 118) states that "societies use psychiatry for the maintenance of cultural and ideological integrity." In response to recent economic and political crises, the ideological role of psychiatry has become even more important in this respect. Certainly, Hickling (2002: 118) believes that following 9/11, "all psychiatry is political psychiatry!" This state of psychiatric hegemony in neoliberal society would appear to make any form of challenge to the ideological state apparatus futile, yet in the following, concluding chapter of this book I will suggest some relatively practical ways in which we can continue to resist the dominant, individualising discourse from the psy-professions.

Bibliography

American Psychiatric Association. (2013) *Diagnostic and Statistical Manual of Mental Disorders* (5th ed.). Arlington, VA: American Psychiatric Association.

Birley, J. L. T. (2000) 'Political Abuse of Psychiatry', *Acta Psychiatrica Scandinavica*, 101(399): 13–15.

Bonnie, R. J. (2002) 'Political Abuse of Psychiatry in the Soviet Union and in China: Complexities and Controversies', *Journal of the American Academy of Psychiatry and the Law*, 30(1): 136–144.

Breggin, P. R. (1993) 'Psychiatry's Role in the Holocaust', *International Journal of Risk & Safety in Medicine*, 4(2): 133–148.

Breggin, P. R., and Breggin, G. R. (1998) *The War Against Children of Color: Psychiatry Targets Inner City Youth*. Monroe: Common Courage Press.

Burleigh, M. (1994) 'Psychiatry, German Society, and the Nazi "Euthanasia" Programme', *Social History of Medicine*, 7(2): 213–228.

Burstow, B. (2015) *Psychiatry and the Business of Madness: An Ethical and Epistemological Accounting*. New York: Palgrave Macmillan.

Cohen, B. M. Z. (2014a) 'Emil Kraepelin', in Scull, A. (Ed.), *Cultural Sociology of Mental Illness: An A-to-Z Guide* (pp. 440–442). Thousand Oaks: Sage.

Cohen, B. M. Z. (2014b) 'Passive-Aggressive: Māori Resistance and the Continuance of Colonial Psychiatry in Aotearoa New Zealand', *Disability and the Global South*, 1(2): 319–339.

Du Bois, W. E. B. (1901) 'The Freedmen's Bureau', *Atlantic Monthly*, 87(519): 354–365.

Fanon, F. (1965) *The Wretched of the Earth*. Harmondsworth: Penguin.

Fernando, S. (2010) *Mental Health, Race and Culture* (3rd ed.). Houndmills, Basingstoke: Palgrave Macmillan.

Foucault, M. (1988b) *Politics, Philosophy, Culture: Interviews and Other Writings, 1977–1984*. Routledge: New York.

Gabbidon, S. L. (2015) *Criminological Perspectives on Race and Crime* (3rd ed.). New York: Routledge.

Galton, F. (1892) *Hereditary Genius: An Inquiry into its Laws and Consequences* (2nd ed.). London: Macmillan.

Gambino, M. (2008) '"These Strangers within Our Gates": Race, Psychiatry and Mental Illness among Black Americans at St Elizabeths Hospital in Washington, DC, 1900–40', *History of Psychiatry*, 19(4): 387–408.

Greenberg, G. (2013) *The Book of Woe: The DSM and The Unmaking of Psychiatry*. New York: Blue Rider Press.

Hassenfeld, I. N. (2002) 'Doctor-Patient Relations in Nazi Germany and the Fate of Psychiatric Patients', *Psychiatric Quarterly*, 73(3): 183–194.

Healey, D. (2014) 'Russian and Soviet Forensic Psychiatry: Troubled and Troubling', *International Journal of Law and Psychiatry*, 37(1): 71–81.

Hickling, F. W. (2002) 'The Political Misuse of Psychiatry: An African-Caribbean Perspective', *Journal of the American Academy of Psychiatry and the Law*, 30(1): 112–119.

Hoffman, D. H., Carter, D. J., Viglucci Lopez, C. R., Benzmiller, H. L., Guo, A. X., Yasir Latifi, S., and Craig, D. C. (2015) *Report to the Special Committee of the Board of Directors of the American Psychological Association: Independent Review Relating to APA Ethics Guidelines, National Security Interrogations, and Torture*. Chicago: Sidley Austin LLP.

Keller, R. C. (2007) *Colonial Madness: Psychiatry in French North Africa*. Chicago: University of Chicago Press.

Kelly, R. (1973) 'Mental Illness in the Māori Population of Aotearoa New Zealand', *Acta Psychiatrica Scandinavica*, 49(6): 722–734.

Keukens, R., and van Voren, R. (2007) 'Coercion in Psychiatry: Still an Instrument of Political Misuse?', *BMC Psychiatry*, 7(1): S4.

Kutchins, H., and Kirk, S. A. (1997) *Making Us Crazy: DSM: The Psychiatric Bible and the Creation of Mental Disorders*. New York: Free Press.

Lee, S., and Kleinman, A. (2002) 'Psychiatry in its Political and Professional Contexts: A Response to Robin Munro', *Journal of the American Academy of Psychiatry and the Law*, 30(1): 120–125.

Lieberman, J. A. (2015) *Shrinks: The Untold Story of Psychiatry*. New York: Little, Brown and Company.

Lifton, R. J. (2000) *The Nazi Doctors: Medical Killing and the Psychology of Genocide* (rev. ed.). New York: Basic Books.

Lombroso, C., Gibson, M., and Rafter, N. H. (2006) *Criminal Man*. Durham: Duke University Press.

Mayer, J. (2009) 'The Secret History: Can Leon Panetta Move the C.I.A. Forward Without Confronting its Past?', *The New Yorker*, http://www.newyorker.com/magazine/2009/06/22/the-secret-history (retrieved on 19 April 2016).

McCallum, D. (2001) *Personality and Dangerousness: Genealogies of Antisocial Personality Disorder*. New York: Cambridge University Press.

McGovern, D., and Cope, R. (1987) 'The Compulsory Detention of Males of Different Ethnic Groups, with Special Reference to Offender Patients', *British Journal of Psychiatry*, 150(4): 505–512.

Metzl, J. (2009) *The Protest Psychosis: How Schizophrenia Became a Black Disease*. Boston: Beacon Press.

Meyer, J-E. (1988) 'The Fate of the Mentally Ill in Germany During the Third Reich', *Psychological Medicine*, 18(3): 575–581.

MindFreedom. (2012) 'MLK on IAACM: Martin Luther King on the International Association for the Advancement of Creative Maladjustment', *MFI*, http://www.mindfreedom.org/kb/mental-health-global/iaacm/MLK-on-IAACM (retrieved on 18 April 2016).

Munro, R. J. (2002) 'Political Psychiatry in Post-Mao China and its Origins in the Cultural Revolution', *Journal of the American Academy of Psychiatry and the Law*, 30(1): 97–106.

Park, Y. S., Park, S. M., Jun, J. Y., and Kim, S. J. (2014) 'Psychiatry in Former Socialist Countries: Implications for North Korean Psychiatry', *Psychiatry Investigation*, 11(4): 363–370.

Parker, I. (2007) *Revolution in Psychology: Alienation to Emancipation*. London: Pluto Press.

Reevy, G. M. (2014) 'Eugenics', in Scull, A. (Ed.), *Cultural Sociology of Mental Illness: An A-to-Z Guide* (pp. 294–296). Thousand Oaks: Sage.

Risen, J. (2014) *Pay Any Price: Greed, Power, and Endless War*. Boston: Houghton Mifflin Harcourt.

Roman, L. G., Brown, S., Noble, S., Wainer, R., and Young, A. E. (2009) 'No Time for Nostalgia!: Asylum-Making, Medicalized Colonialism in British Columbia (1859–97) and Artistic Praxis for Social Transformation', *International Journal of Qualitative Studies in Education*, 22(1): 17–63.

Scull, A. (1984) *Decarceration: Community Treatment and the Deviant: A Radical View* (2nd ed.). Oxford: Basil Blackwell.

Seeman, M. V. (2005) 'Psychiatry in the Nazi Era', *Canadian Journal of Psychiatry*, 50(4): 218–225.

Shorter, E. (1997) *A History of Psychiatry: From the Era of the Asylum to the Age of Prozac*. New York: John Wiley & Sons.

Stone, A. A. (2002) 'Psychiatrists on the Side of the Angels: The Falun Gong and Soviet Jewry', *Journal of the American Academy of Psychiatry and the Law*, 30(1): 107–111.

Strous, R. D. (2006) 'Nazi Euthanasia of the Mentally Ill at Hadamar', *American Journal of Psychiatry*, 163(1): 27.

Strous, R. D. (2007) 'Psychiatry During the Nazi Era: Ethical Lessons for the Modern Professional', *Annals of General Psychiatry*, 6(1), doi:10.1186/1744-859X-6-8.

Szasz, T. S. (1988) *Schizophrenia: The Sacred Symbol of Psychiatry*. Syracuse: Syracuse University Press.

Tseris, E. (2013) 'Trauma Theory Without Feminism? Evaluating Contemporary Understandings of Traumatized Women', *Affilia: Journal of Women and Social Work*, 28(2): 153–164.

van Voren, R. (2002) 'Comparing Soviet and Chinese Political Psychiatry', *Journal of the American Academy of Psychiatry and the Law Online*, 30(1): 131–135.

van Voren, R. (2010) 'Political Abuse of Psychiatry-An Historical Overview', *Schizophrenia Bulletin*, 36(1): 33–35.

Vaughan, M. (2007) 'Introduction', in S. Mahone, and M. Vaughan (Eds.), *Psychiatry and Empire* (pp. 1–16). Houndmills, Basingstoke: Palgrave Macmillan.

von Cranach, M. (2010) 'Ethics in Psychiatry: The Lessons We Learn from Nazi Psychiatry', *European Archives of Psychiatry and Clinical Neuroscience*, 260(2): S152–S156.

Walker, R. (1990) *Ka Whawhai Tonu Matou Struggle Without End.* Auckland: Penguin.

Welch, M. (2010) 'Illusions in Truth Seeking: The Perils of Interrogation and Torture in the War on Terror', *Social Justice*, 37(2/3): 123–148.

Zimbardo, P. G. (2002) 'Psychology in the Public Service', *American Psychologist*, 57(6/7): 431–433.

8

Conclusion: Challenging the Psychiatric Hegemon

This book has developed a Marxist argument for understanding psychiatry and allied professions as agents of social control which serve capitalist prerogatives. Rather than concerned with the health of the population, I have drawn on extensive evidence to argue that the psy-professions were created and progressed to regulate and manage western populations through personalising social and economic issues, pathologising political dissent, policing and punishing problematic and deviant groups, and reproducing the dominant norms and values of the ruling elite through psychiatric discourse. Even if readers do not entirely accept my position, I hope I have by now convinced them that the mental health system is a fundamentally political project.

To briefly recap the main issues with the psychiatric knowledge base: there is still no proof for any "mental illness" produced by the psychiatric discourse, and given this state of affairs it is unsurprising that psychiatrists cannot prove causation (biological or otherwise) for such "disease," or that any of their "treatments" for mental pathology (including ECT, drugs, and therapy) "work." Psychiatrists still cannot accurately determine who is "mentally ill" and who is "mentally healthy." Rather than fixed social realities, psychiatric labels such as homosexuality, gender

B.M.Z. Cohen, *Psychiatric Hegemony*,
DOI 10.1057/978-1-137-46051-6_8

dysphoria, hysteria, ADHD, drapetomania, borderline personality disorder, and masturbatory insanity are historically and culturally contingent.

Further, the previous chapters have outlined some of the many atrocities committed by the psy-professionals as part of their moral management of non-complaint and deviant populations. This has included the normalisation of conditions of slavery, the psychiatric incarceration of political activists, the labelling and drugging of young people with school-related "disorders," the lobotomising of problematic wives, the torture of war combatants, the castration of working class men and women, the pathologisation of the unemployed, and the mass murder of psychiatric inmates. Thus, as agents of social control, the psy-professionals have been responsible for maintaining the status quo under the guise of a neutral and scientific authority on "mental health."

Notwithstanding all of these problems, the psy-professions have thrived over the past 35 years. This is not due to any success in accurately identifying, treating or "curing" mental disease—rates of "mental illness" have increased dramatically while "curability" is seldom even mentioned as an aim for the mental health "experts" anymore—but rather the requirements of neoliberalism. The fluidity of the psychiatric discourse has proved valuable to capitalism in producing medical diagnoses that mirror dominant economic and ideological codes. As I have argued in this book, neoliberalism's focus on individual competition, personal responsibility, and the self as the site of change is a perfect fit with knowledge claims on "mental illness" which promote self-surveillance and the individual's monitoring of "risky behaviour." Through detailed socio-historical analyses of the emergence of some of the current diagnostic categories of "mental illness" such as SAD, ADHD, and BPD I have demonstrated in this book how the psychiatric discourse of the psy-professionals has become hegemonic in neoliberal society. The requirement of the ruling classes to govern at a distance and the necessity to reinforce and reproduce the dominant norms and values of late capitalism in many more arenas of public and private life have allowed practices, treatments, and the assertions of "mental health" workers to expand beyond the psychiatric institution into, among other places, unemployment offices, prisons, educational and training facilities, the military, the workplace, and our homes.

As the current or future victims of the psychiatric discourse, this chapter briefly discusses two ways in which we can move towards the abolition of the ideological state apparatus which encompasses psychiatry and its many allies. The route to abolition of this oppressive order is of course far from straightforward. My Marxist argument necessarily entails the end of capitalism, yet there is also plenty that can be done to subdue and diminish psy-power before the current economic order finally collapses. This involves the disruption of the psychiatric discourse on many fronts through an alliance of political activists on the left, psychiatric survivors, critical and radical academics and students, and community leaders.

Towards Abolition

Despite facing greater levels of social and economic hardship, there is a good reason why people in low-income countries experience less mental illness and have more chance of long-term recovery than their counterparts in higher income countries (Whitaker 2010b: 227–228). Namely, they have little or no access to western-trained mental health experts who can readily pathologise their behaviour as signs of mental disease. Lest we forget, there are societies that live perfectly happy (in fact, happier) without psychiatrists, psychologists, therapists, counsellors, life coaches, and agony aunts and uncles. Meanwhile, we in the west are recipients of a failed psychiatric enterprise in which the amount of "mental illness" continues to increase, not due to any real health epidemic but rather as a form of medicalised social control at the instigation of neoliberal capital. This is why, in the words of Burstow (2015: 229), "the institution of psychiatry must go." And with it, I would add that all the allied professions associated with dictating and controlling our behaviour through the psychiatric discourse must also go.

As Masson (1994: 316) has stated, "[p]sychiatry has not distinguished itself by fighting in the front lines for social justice and against human oppression. It is time this fact was recognised and the implications drawn." The psy-professions are not on our side, they have never stood up for us. In fact, quite the reverse. As we have seen in this book, the class interests of the psy-professions closely align with the ruling elites, so it is no surprise that their knowledge claims on mental health and illness support the status quo. As Roberts (2015: 6) has recently stated of the production of "facts" on pathology from the psychological sciences, "[t]hese are arrived at outside the scientific arena and then imported into it by a system of smoke and mirrors to claim scientific backing for what are essentially political or moral judgments." Thus, despite having some psy-professional friends and colleagues whom I continue to work with on various research projects, I would at this stage be a fool to recommend anything other than the wholesale abolition of their profession. This is the logical conclusion from my research and theoretical argumentation in the book.

There are a few practical things that can be done immediately to challenge and weaken the power of the psy-professions. As they maintain the ultimate power in defining, measuring, and treating "mental disorders," we need to primarily concentrate on the psychiatric profession. Firstly, we must remove psychiatry's compulsory powers. This includes the power to incarcerate and to enforce shock treatment and drugs—including the use of compulsory treatment orders outside the institution, a move which has only served to extend the policing powers of the mental health system—on people against their will. Even if we were to still believe in the work of psychiatry, how can incarceration and torture be a part of any modern system of health care? The psychiatric profession is the only profession with the power to imprison people involuntarily apart from the police; these physical forms of oppression have to end. Secondly, the prescribing rights of the profession should be withdrawn. As we have seen in the book, though drugs do not "work" in the manner psychiatrists would have us believe, they have advantages over insulin therapy, prefrontal lobotomies, and ECT. Namely, they are cheaper, and the dangers of usage are generally less noticeable in the short term. As western countries are slowly moving towards the decriminalisation of illegal drugs, it makes sense that the drugs which have previously been known as "anti-psychotics" or "antidepressants"—highly misleading terminology—are also independently tested for toxicity and then accurately labelled for potential over-the-counter sales. Despite being no more effective than placebo, I know that some people still find these drugs useful: some feel they are calmer while others have stated that the pills give them more confidence. Relatively unrestricted access to drugs that include an accurate warning on the increased risk of an early death is always preferable to their control by psychiatrists who use prescription rights to claim medical expertise and authority on "mental illness."

It is long overdue, but thirdly, ECT needs to be outlawed. As I have discussed in the book, not only is shock treatment still being inflicted on "hard to reach" cases when the drugs "fail" (meaning the inmate is not subdued to the psychiatrist's satisfaction), it is actually experiencing a revival, with uncooperative women again being a major target. Soon psychosurgery will be back with us. The only demonstrable effects of ECT to date have been memory loss, brain damage, and a heightened chance of suicide. ECT machinery should be in a museum of horrors, not used in health practice. We must collectively agitate and protest to have ECT banned. The group ECT Justice! is one of a number calling for the elimination of ECT; it has good online resources and regularly coordinates global action and protests against the use of such "treatment"(see http://www.ectjustice.com/index.php).

In working towards the abolition of the psy-professions, it is also necessary to form closer alliances between academics, left wing activists, community groups, and progressive psychiatric survivor organisations. During the writing of this book, I was emailed by a psychiatric survivor in the United States who pointed out that my Marxist arguments on psychiatric power were far from new; in fact, he stated, psychiatric survivor groups in the 1960s—such as the Psychiatric Inmates/Mental Patients Liberation Movement—were all too well aware of the need to frame the oppressive practices of psychiatry within a broader understanding of capitalist economics and the ideological control of deviant populations (see, e.g., Chamberlin 1990). The spirit of these highly politicised survivor groups continues through independent organisations such as MindFreedom International (see http://www.mindfreedom.org) who campaign against a wide range of oppressive practices carried out by the psy-professions including the use of psychiatric labels and compulsory treatment. Local campaigns—including public protests and non-violent occupations of APA meetings—involve a range of participants including survivors, family members, community groups, political activists, and academics. It is a good example of an organisation which has successfully formed a broad-based alliance with like-minded groups. At the same time, critical scholars should be prepared to take the lead in facilitating local activism through the institutional hosting and resourcing of specific events; these can in turn act as a catalyst for future protests and campaigns against the mental health system (for a good example, see the Mad Studies Network, https://madstudies2014.wordpress.com).

Challenging the Apologists

As neoliberalism has infected higher education, research on "mental health issues" in the academy has become increasingly conservative. My own subject area, sociology, is as guilty as any other. We have lost sight of what it means to think critically about the mental health system, to be able to challenge the work of the psy-professions, to interrogate meaningfully the production of knowledge claims on "mental disease," and to adequately contextualise the expansion of the psychiatric discourse with reference to theoretical sets of ideas which refer to labelling, power, and social control. We have effectively become pseudo-social psychologists whose research agenda is passed down to us by state agencies, requiring us to do little more than identify marginalised groups who can be labelled and policed by the psychiatric authorities and the criminal justice system. Having a once proud tradition of highlighting the systematic, oppressive practices of the mental health system, the sociology of mental health is now in severe danger of simply becoming another arm of the state. Far too much of what passes for "research" in the discipline is flawed from the beginning: it takes for granted that the mental health system is a fundamentally caring, scientifically sound discipline; it accepts mental illness diagnoses as valid and having a proved aetiology; and the empirical lens is focused outward on "undetected" pathologies in the general population rather than inward on the pathological behaviour of the institution of psychiatry and its allies. The result is that we end up with sociological research and scholarship which perpetuates the myths of psychiatric knowledge and aids the expansion of psychiatric hegemony (how many times have we read at the conclusion of such articles and books that there is a gap—an "unmet need"—in current mental health provision for which further resources and staffing is required?).

Thus, we need to resist the top-down state-run agenda and reject funding streams that tie us into conservative, surveillance-focused projects. We also need to be vocal in challenging the scholars who take on such projects and reproduce the same old nonsense on mental illness prevalence which reinforces the hegemonic view of black, female, young, LGBT, working class, and other marginalised populations as pathological. As always, sociological investigation needs to focus on the powerful rather than the powerless. This requires the revitalisation of a truly critical research agenda for the sociology of mental health in which the operations and practices of the psy-professions and their production of knowledge claims are prioritised. Research would then focus on the politics of diagnostic construction and professional power, on how psy-professionals turn subjective, personal understandings of human beings into categories of pathology, on the inner workings of the mental health system, on the conflicts and alliances made internally and externally to these professions, and on their constant need to justify mental health practice as medically and scientifically relevant.

Alongside producing a critical research agenda, we need to revitalise social theory within the analysis of such research. The amount of theory-free scholarship on mental health and illness currently in circulation is of grave concern to the future of general critical investigation within the academy. We are failing in our public duty as the critic and conscience of society if we cannot frame research findings beyond immediate experience. Encouraging our students and our colleagues to think critically about their research necessarily involves a grounding in theoretical sets of ideas on the world, in understanding social and economic forces which inhibit or emancipate certain groups, the power imbalances which exist in certain societies, and the production and privileging of certain forms of knowledge over others in capitalism. Within this, critical theories on mental health and illness need to be prioritised—rather than marginalised—in the sociology of mental health. Towards this specific aim, my next book is a long-overdue collection of original works from scholars who continue to engage with critical perspectives in the area (see Cohen, forthcoming). I hope that this work will lead to an extended dialogue on critical research and theoretical developments for those working within—as well as outside—the academy.

Bibliography

Burstow, B. (2015) *Psychiatry and the Business of Madness: An Ethical and Epistemological Accounting*. New York: Palgrave Macmillan.

Chamberlin, J. (1990) 'The Ex-Patients' Movement: Where We've Been and Where We're Going', *Journal of Mind and Behavior*, 11(3): 323–336.

Cohen, B. M. Z. (ed.) (forthcoming) *Routledge International Handbook of Critical Mental Health*. Abingdon: Routledge.

Masson, J. M. (1994) *Against Therapy* (rev. ed.). Monroe: Common Courage Press.

Roberts, R. (2015) *Psychology and Capitalism: The Manipulation of Mind*. Alresford: Zero Books.

Whitaker, R. (2010b) *Mad in America: Bad Science, Bad Medicine, and the Enduring Mistreatment of the Mentally Ill* (rev. ed.) New York: Basic Books.

Appendix A: Methodology for Textual Analysis of the DSMs

Using the "advanced search" tool for PDF files in Adobe Acrobat Reader, word searches on each edition of the DSM were conducted by a research assistant (Rearna Hartmann; hereafter, RH) using pre-designated keywords provided by the author. From the instances in which the word was highlighted, RH checked that the word, first, was used in the correct context and, second, occurred in the main body of the manual (i.e., within the mental illness classifications themselves rather than the front- or end-matter). In cases where it was not possible for RH to individually check each instance of the word, she developed a few methods of elimination of word counts by checking for key phrases in which a word appeared outside of the intended context (e.g., "play a role" occurred multiple times when searching for the word "play"). In these cases, the number of times those phrases occurred was subtracted from the main word count. RH also subtracted any words that were counted in the file that were not in the main text. This was done by utilising the word search tool which gives each occurrence of the word according to where it appears in the text, then using the page numbers provided in the DSM's table of contents and subtracting all the occurrences that were either in the references or preamble to the main text.

B.M.Z. Cohen, *Psychiatric Hegemony*,
DOI 10.1057/978-1-137-46051-6

Appendix B: Youth-Related Diagnostic Categories in the DSM, 1952–2013

DSM-I (1952)	Adjustment reaction of adolescence (p. 42) Adjustment reaction of childhood (p. 41) Adjustment reaction of infancy (p. 41) Conduct disturbance (p. 41) Schizophrenic reaction, childhood type (p. 6) Special symptom reaction, enuresis (p. 39) Special symptom reaction, learning disturbance (p. 39) Special symptom reaction, speech disturbance (p. 39)
DSM-II (1968)	Adjustment reaction of adolescence (p. 49) Adjustment reaction of childhood (p. 49) Adjustment reaction of infancy (p. 49) Group delinquent reaction of childhood (or adolescence) (p. 51) Hyperkinetic reaction of childhood (or adolescence) (p. 50) Mental retardation (p. 14) Overanxious reaction of childhood (or adolescence) (p. 50) Runaway reaction of childhood (or adolescence) (p. 50) Schizophrenia, childhood type (p. 35) Special symptoms, disorder of sleep (p. 48) Special symptoms, encopresis (p. 48) Special symptoms, enuresis (p. 48) Special symptoms, feeding disturbance (p. 48) Special symptoms, specific learning disturbance (p. 48) Special symptoms, speech disturbance (p. 48) Special symptoms, tic (p. 48) Unsocialized aggressive reaction of childhood (or adolescence) (p. 50) Withdrawing reaction of childhood (or adolescence) (p. 50)

(*continued*)

B.M.Z. Cohen, *Psychiatric Hegemony*,
DOI 10.1057/978-1-137-46051-6

Appendix B (continued)

DSM-III (1980)	Adjustment disorder with disturbance of conduct (p. 301) Attention deficit disorder (p. 41) Atypical specific developmental disorder (p. 99) Atypical stereotyped movement disorder (p. 77) Atypical tic disorder (p. 77) Avoidant disorder of childhood or adolescence (p. 53) Chronic motor tic disorder (p. 75) Conduct disorder (p. 45): – atypical – socialized, aggressive – socialized, non-aggressive – undersocialized, aggressive – undersocialized, non-aggressive Developmental arithmetic disorder (p. 94) Developmental articulation disorder (p. 98) Developmental language disorder (p. 95) Developmental reading disorder (p. 93) Elective mutism (p. 62) Functional encopresis (p. 81) Functional enuresis (p. 79) Gender identity disorder of childhood (p. 264) Identity disorder (p. 65) Infantile autism (p. 87) Kleptomania (p. 293) Mental retardation (p. 36) Mixed specific developmental disorder (p. 98) Oppositional disorder (p. 63) Pica (p. 71) Pyromania (p. 294) Reactive attachment disorder of infancy (p. 57) Rumination disorder of infancy (p. 72) Schizoid disorder of childhood or adolescence (p. 60) Separation anxiety disorder (p. 50) Sleep terror disorder (p. 84) Stuttering (p. 78) Tourette's disorder (p. 76) Transient tic disorder (p. 74)

(continued)

Appendix B (continued)

DSM-III-R (1987)	Adjustment disorder with disturbance of conduct (p. 329) Adjustment disorder with work (or academic) Inhibition (p. 329) Attention-deficit hyperactivity disorder (p. 50) Autistic disorder (p. 38) Avoidant disorder of childhood or adolescence (p. 61) Chronic motor or vocal tic disorder (p. 81) Cluttering (p. 85) Conduct disorder (p. 53): – group type – solitary aggressive type – undifferentiated type Developmental arithmetic disorder (p. 41) Developmental articulation disorder (p. 44) Developmental coordination disorder (p. 48) Developmental expressive language disorder (p. 45) Developmental expressive writing disorder (p. 42) Developmental reading disorder (p. 43) Developmental receptive language disorder (p. 47) Dream anxiety disorder (nightmare disorder) (p. 308) Elective mutism (p. 88) Functional encopresis (p. 82) Functional enuresis (p. 84) Gender identity disorder of childhood (p. 71) Identity disorder (p. 89) Kleptomania (p. 322) Mental retardation (p. 28) Oppositional defiant disorder (p. 56) Overanxious disorder (p. 63) Pathological gambling (p. 324) Pervasive developmental disorder not otherwise specified (p. 39) Pica (p. 69) Pyromania (p. 325) Reactive attachment disorder of infancy or early childhood (p. 91) Rumination disorder of infancy (p. 70) Separation anxiety disorder (p. 58) Sleep terror disorder (p. 310) Stereotypy/habit disorder (p. 93) Stuttering (p. 86) Tourette's disorder (p. 79) Transient tic disorder (p. 81) Undifferentiated attention deficit disorder (p. 95)

(*continued*)

Appendix B (continued)

DSM-IV (1994)	Adjustment disorder with disturbance of conduct (p. 623) Asperger's disorder (p. 75) Attention-deficit/hyperactivity disorder (p. 78) Autistic disorder (p. 66) Childhood disintegrative disorder (p. 73) Chronic motor or vocal tic disorder (p. 103) Communication disorder not otherwise specified (p. 65) Conduct disorder (p. 85): – adolescent-onset type – childhood-onset type Dependent personality disorder (p. 665) Developmental coordination disorder (p. 53) Disorder of written expression (p. 51) Disruptive behavior disorder not otherwise specified (p. 94) Encopresis (p. 106) Enuresis (p. 108) Expressive language disorder (p. 55) Feeding disorder of infancy or early childhood (p. 98) Gender identity disorder in children (p. 532) Kleptomania (612) Learning disorder not otherwise specified (p. 53) Mathematics disorder (p. 50) Mental retardation (p. 39) Mixed receptive–expressive language disorder (p. 58) Nightmare disorder (p. 580) Oppositional defiant disorder (p. 91) Paranoid personality disorder (p. 636) Pervasive developmental disorder not otherwise specified (p. 77) Phonological disorder (p. 61) Pyromania (p. 614) Pica (p. 95) Reactive attachment disorder of infancy or early childhood (p. 116) Reading disorder (p. 48) Rett's disorder (p. 71) Rumination disorder (p. 96) Selective mutism (p. 114) Separation anxiety disorder (p. 110) Sleep terror disorder (p. 583) Stereotypic movement disorder (p. 118) Stuttering (p. 63) Tourette's disorder (p. 101) Transient tic disorder (p. 104)

(continued)

Appendix B (continued)

DSM-IV-TR (2000)	Adjustment disorder with disturbance of conduct (p. 679) Asperger's disorder (p. 80) Attention-deficit/hyperactivity disorder (p. 85) Attention-deficit/hyperactivity disorder not otherwise specified (p. 93) Autistic disorder (p. 70) Childhood disintegrative disorder (p. 77) Chronic motor or vocal tic disorder (p. 114) Communication disorder not otherwise specified (p. 69) Conduct disorder (p. 93): – adolescent-onset type – childhood-onset type – unspecified onset Developmental coordination disorder (p. 56) Disorder of written expression (p. 54) Disruptive behavior disorder not otherwise specified (p. 103) Encopresis (p. 116) Enuresis (p. 118) Expressive language disorder (p. 58) Feeding disorder of infancy or early childhood (p. 107) Gender identity disorder in children (p. 576) Kleptomania (p. 667) Learning disorder not otherwise specified (p. 56) Mathematics disorder (p. 53) Mental retardation (p. 41) Mixed receptive-expressive language disorder (p. 62) Nightmare disorder (p. 631) Oppositional defiant disorder (p. 100) Pervasive developmental disorder not otherwise specified (p. 84) Phonological disorder (p. 65) Pica (p. 103) Pyromania (p. 669) Reactive attachment disorder of infancy or early childhood (p. 127) Reading disorder (p. 51) Rett's disorder (p. 760) Rumination disorder (p. 105) Selective mutism (p. 125) Separation anxiety disorder (p. 121) Sleep terror disorder (p. 634) Stereotypic movement disorder (p. 131) Stuttering (p. 67) Tic disorder not otherwise specified (p. 116) Tourette's disorder (p. 111) Transient tic disorder (p. 115)

(*continued*)

Appendix B (continued)

DSM-5 (2013)	Adjustment disorder with disturbance of conduct (p. 286) Attention-deficit/hyperactivity disorder (p. 59) Autism spectrum disorder (p. 50) Childhood-onset fluency disorder (stuttering) (p. 45) Conduct disorder (p. 469) Developmental coordination disorder (p. 74) Disinhibited social engagement disorder (p. 268) Encopresis (p. 357) Enuresis (p. 355) Gender dysphoria in children (p. 452) Global developmental delay (p. 41) Intellectual disability (intellectual developmental disorder) (p. 33) Internet gaming disorder (p. 795) Kleptomania (p. 478) Language disorder (p. 42) Nightmare disorder (p. 404) Non-rapid eye movement sleep arousal disorders, sleep terror type (p. 399) Oppositional defiant disorder (p. 462) Other specified attention-deficit/hyperactivity disorder (p. 65) Other specified disruptive, impulse-control, and conduct disorder (p. 479) Other specified elimination disorder (p. 359) Other specified neurodevelopmental disorder (p. 86) Other specified tic disorder (p. 85) Persistent (chronic) motor or vocal tic disorder (p. 81) Pica (p. 329) Post-traumatic stress disorder (p. 271) Provisional tic disorder (p. 81) Pyromania (p. 476) Reactive attachment disorder (p. 265) Rumination disorder (p. 332) Selective mutism (p. 195) Separation anxiety disorder (p. 190) Social (pragmatic) communication disorder (p. 47) Specific learning disorder (p. 66): – with impairment in mathematics – with impairment in reading – with impairment in written expression Speech sound disorder (p. 44) Stereotypic movement disorder (p. 77) Tourette's disorder (p. 81) Unspecified attention-deficit/hyperactivity disorder (p. 66) Unspecified communication disorder (p. 49) Unspecified disruptive, impulse-control, and conduct disorder (p. 480) Unspecified elimination disorder (p. 360) Unspecified intellectual disability (intellectual developmental disorder) (p. 41) Unspecified neurodevelopmental disorder (p. 86) Unspecified tic disorder (p. 85)

Appendix C: "Feminised" Diagnostic Categories in the DSM, 1952–2013

DSM-I (1952)	Homosexuality (p. 121)
	Manic-depressive reaction, manic type (p. 25)
	Psychotic depressive reaction (p. 25)
	Sexual deviation (p. 38)
DSM-II (1968)	Anxiety neurosis (p. 39)
	Depressive neurosis (p. 40)
	Homosexuality (p. 44)
	Hysterical neurosis (p. 39)
	Hysterical personality (p. 43)
	Manic-depressive illness, manic type (p. 36)
	Obsessive-compulsive neurosis (p. 40)
	Psychosis with childbirth (p. 31)
	Transvestitism (p. 44)
DSM-III (1980)	Agoraphobia without panic attacks (p. 226)
	Agoraphobia with panic attacks (p. 226)
	Anorexia nervosa (p. 67)
	Atypical somatoform disorder (p. 251)
	Borderline personality disorder (p. 321)
	Bulimia (p. 69)
	Conversion disorder (or hysterical neurosis, conversion type) (p. 244)
	Cyclothymic disorder (p. 218)
	Dependent personality disorder (p. 324)
	Dysthymic disorder (or depressive neurosis) (p. 220)
	Ego-dystonic homosexuality (p. 282)
	Functional vaginismus (p. 280)
	Generalized anxiety disorder (p. 232)
	Histrionic personality disorder (p. 313)
	Inhibited female orgasm (p. 279)
	Panic disorder (p. 230)
	Post-traumatic stress disorder (p. 236)
	Somatization disorder (p. 240)
	Transvestism (p. 269)

(*continued*)

B.M.Z. Cohen, *Psychiatric Hegemony*,
DOI 10.1057/978-1-137-46051-6

Appendix C (continued)

DSM-III-R (1987)	Agoraphobia without history of panic disorder (p. 240) Bipolar disorder (p. 225) Body dysmorphic disorder (p. 255) Borderline personality disorder (p. 347) Conversion disorder (or hysterical neurosis, conversion type) (p. 257) Dependent personality disorder (p. 353) Dysthymia (or depressive neurosis) (p. 230) Female sexual arousal disorder (p. 294) Gender identity disorder of adolescence or adulthood, nontranssexual type (p. 76) Generalized anxiety disorder (p. 251) Histrionic personality disorder (p. 348) Inhibited female orgasm (p. 294) Panic disorder with agoraphobia (p. 235) Transsexualism (p. 74) Transvestic fetishism (p. 288) Vaginismus (p. 295)
DSM-IV (1994)	Anorexia nervosa (p. 539) Body dysmorphic disorder (p. 466) Borderline personality disorder (p. 650) Bulimia nervosa (p. 545) Dependent personality disorder (p. 665) Dysthymic disorder (p. 345) Eating disorder not otherwise specified (p. 550) Female dyspareunia due to ... (indicate the general medical condition) (p. 515) Female hypoactive sexual desire disorder due to ... (indicate the general medical condition) (p. 515) Female orgasmic disorder (p. 505) Female sexual arousal disorder (p. 500) Gender identity disorder (p. 532) Generalized anxiety disorder (p. 432) Histrionic personality disorder (p. 655) Other female sexual dysfunction due to ... (indicate the general medical condition) (p. 515) Panic disorder with agoraphobia (p. 397) Post-traumatic stress disorder (p. 424) Sedative, hypnotic, or anxiolytic abuse (p. 263) Somatization disorder (p. 446) Transvestic fetishism (p. 530) Vaginismus (p. 513)

(*continued*)

Appendix C (continued)

DSM-IV-TR (2000)	Anorexia nervosa (p. 583) Binge-eating disorder (p. 785) Body dysmorphic disorder (p. 507) Borderline personality disorder (p. 706) Bulimia nervosa (p. 589) Dependent personality disorder (p. 721) Dysthymic disorder (p. 376) Eating disorder not otherwise specified (p. 594) Female dyspareunia due to ... (indicate the general medical condition) (p. 558) Female hypoactive sexual desire disorder due to ... (indicate the general medical condition) (p. 558) Female orgasmic disorder (p. 547) Female sexual arousal disorder (p. 543) Gender identity disorder (p. 576) Gender identity disorder not otherwise specified (p. 582) Generalized anxiety disorder (p. 472) Histrionic personality disorder (p. 711) Other female sexual dysfunction due to ... (indicate the general medical condition) (p. 558) Panic disorder with agoraphobia (p. 433) Post-partum onset specifier (p. 422) Post-traumatic stress disorder (p. 463) Premenstrual dysphoric disorder (p. 381) Sedative, hypnotic, or anxiolytic abuse (p. 268) Somatization disorder (p. 486) Transvestic fetishism (p. 574) Vaginismus (not due to a general medical condition) (p. 556)
DSM-5 (2013)	Acute stress disorder (p. 280) Agoraphobia (p. 217) Anorexia nervosa (p. 338) Avoidant/restrictive food intake disorder (p. 334) Binge-eating disorder (p. 350) Body dysmorphic disorder (p. 242) Borderline personality disorder (p. 663) Bulimia nervosa (p. 345) Conversion disorder (p. 318) Dependent personality disorder (p. 675) Female orgasmic disorder (p. 429) Female sexual interest/arousal disorder (p. 432) Gender dysphoria (p. 451) Generalized anxiety disorder (p. 222) Genito-pelvic pain/penetration disorder (p. 437) Histrionic personality disorder (p. 667) Other specified feeding or eating disorder (p. 353) Other specified gender dysphoria (p. 459) Post-traumatic stress disorder (p. 271) Premenstrual dysphoric disorder (p. 171) Somatic symptom disorder (p. 311) Transvestic disorder, with fetishism, with autogynephilia (p. 702) Unspecified feeding or eating disorder (p. 354) Unspecified gender dysphoria (p. 459)

Index

B.M.Z. Cohen, *Psychiatric Hegemony*,
DOI 10.1057/978-1-137-46051-6

N

Printed by Printforce, the Netherlands